I0104792

From OUCH to "Aaah!"

Second Edition

Thank you so much for purchasing From Ouch to Aaah! Shoulder Pain Self-Care!
There's a free thank you gift waiting for you at:
www.massagepublications.com/ouch-to-aaah-free-gift/

"It takes as much energy to wish as it does to plan."
Eleanor Roosevelt

Disclaimer:
Shoulder problems can be complex, multidimensional and multifaceted. This book is not a comprehensive study of those issues. This book is for educational purposes only and should not be considered a substitute for proper training. It is sold with the understanding that the author and publisher are not engaged in rendering medical or other professional services. If medical advice or other expert assistance is required, the services of an appropriate professional should be sought. Information in this book should not be used to diagnose, treat, or prescribe. The author and publisher shall not be held liable for any damages in connection with, or arising out of anyone's interpretation or application of the information in this manual. The user is encouraged to always use sound judgment in making decisions about her/his ability to perform the exercises.

ACKNOWLEDGEMENTS:
Profound gratitude to those who helped me birth this project:
Frank Kroncke
Suzanne Rittenbury
Keith Fail
Mary Reynolds
Hope Malkan
Patricia Guy
David Dennis
Beverly Voss

Table of Contents

It's the PITS to have shoulder pain!

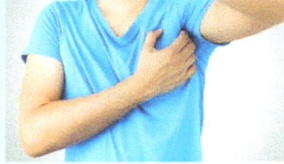

A number of years ago I injured my left rotator cuff during a yoga class. We were doing several poses that required the upper body to bear weight. My injury primarily involved tendonitis of the rotator cuff muscles. Even though my injury would fall into the mild to moderate category it took more than a year to heal. If I had known what I know now, it certainly would have healed much faster. The cause of my injury was not a trauma or blow to my shoulder but incorrect shoulder mechanics. This was a piece of humble pie to swallow since I teach body mechanics, workshops in many massage therapy related subjects, dance and yoga classes!

I went to fellow massage therapists for treatments, which helped, but I was disappointed that none of them educated me about shoulder mechanics. I devoured everything I could read about the shoulder and the rotator cuff and started my own rehabilitation which included strength training, stretching, massage, chiropractic and acupuncture. I even became a personal trainer.

From my research and clinical experience, I've discovered that 90% of all shoulder pain/rotator cuff dysfunctions stem from incorrect shoulder mechanics and are easily preventable.

A common and all too prevalent example of this is sitting slumped at our computers with our shoulders rolled forward.

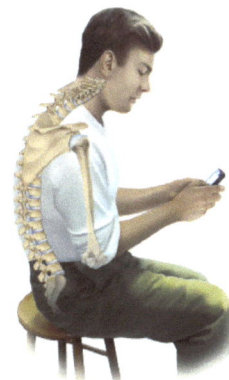

Since then I have seen hundreds of clients with rotator cuff injuries. I believe we can give the best treatments when we have the "inside scoop" on a condition from our own healing journeys. I was inspired to write a book and create a DVD for massage therapists on this subject. Additionally, I have taught my techniques and protocols to thousands of massage therapists across the country. I'm on a mission to create world peace one shoulder at a time!

Often doctors will diagnose shoulder pain as bursitis or arthritis when the real problem is in the rotator cuff. Anti-inflammatory drugs are often prescribed which treats the symptoms but not the cause. Also, doctors may not make the patient aware that a simple change in sleeping position can be profoundly effective. My injury took a significant turn for the better when I changed from sleeping on my left affected side to sleeping on my right side.

One client of mine was given an anti-inflammatory and sent to physical therapy where they prescribed strength training right away. She got worse and then her other shoulder began bothering her. It was too soon for her to do strength training; restoration of a normal soft tissue environment through massage and stretching should have come before working with resistance. There are some first-rate physical therapy clinics and doctors but, unfortunately, there are some bad apples too.

I had another client with shoulder pain who is wheel-chair bound and had a radical mastectomy many years ago. The combination of constantly sitting in a wheel-chair and having a mastectomy has deformed the connective tissue around her right chest to such a degree that the head of her right humerus has a sustained internal pull[+] on it. She had terrible pain in her shoulder. The simple suggestion of sleeping with her shoulders off her pillow (she sleeps on her back) reduced her pain by about 75 percent. Sleeping with her shoulders on the pillow subjected her poor shoulder to even more internal rotation. No wonder she was in such agony! Yet her doctor diagnosed it as arthritis and only increased her pain medication.

I believe that client education (and cooperation) is the key to healing a shoulder/rotator cuff injury. This book is a result of my research into rotator cuff injuries, my clinical experience and teaching continuing education classes on the subject. It reflects my views* on the best way to treat these injuries non-surgically.

This book is intended for mild to moderate injuries and improper use conditions. Anything more serious must be assessed by an osteopath, orthopedic specialist or chiropractor.

Students, clients and colleagues have made valuable suggestions to this book. All inaccuracies are mine alone.

Signs
and
Symptoms
of an
Injured
Rotator
Cuff

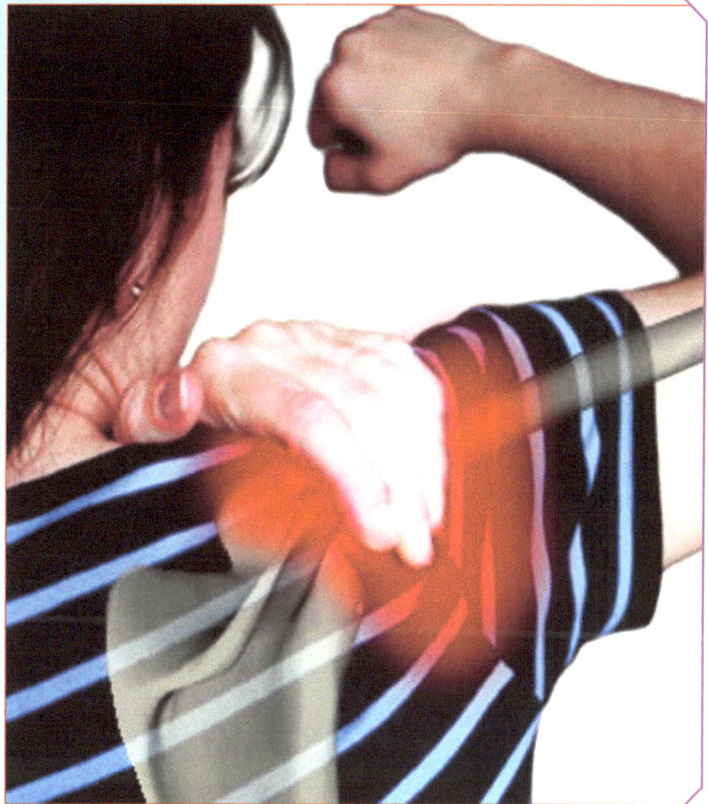

DO YOU HAVE SOME OF THE SIGNS
AND SYMPTOMS OF AN INJURED ROTATOR CUFF?

Problems in the rotator cuff can manifest a variety of symptoms. Remember, all pain in the shoulder has something to do with the rotator cuff, either directly or indirectly. Here's a partial list of the most common signs and symptoms:

• Limited range of motion in the arm/shoulder.

• Pain in the upper arm where the deltoid muscle is, especially when the arm is lifted away from the side in abduction. It may feel like the pain is deep in the shoulder joint. This pain is often from *trigger points* in the rotator cuff muscles.

• Pain at rest or during movement.

• Pain during movements like those involved in getting dressed, brushing hair, reaching back to a night-stand, fastening a seat belt, putting on a coat and many more.

• Weakness in the shoulder.

• A clicking or popping sound when moving the arm.

• A painful arc through part of the range of motion involved in raising your arm above your head. This means you can move your arm without pain up to a certain point; then it hurts for a bit; then the pain goes away. This is called a painful arc.

Do you recognize any of your symptoms? If so, the good news is that your pain can be completely alleviated by this self-care program. Read these testimonials from people just like you with shoulder injuries:

Old jocks like me hate to see the doctor. They rarely have a simple and non-invasive suggestion when I whine about getting old and "My knee's killing me!" or "My shoulder gets this pain. See doc, I once was a great basketball center." Sure, the Glory Days! Now it's a magic pill or two and/or scheduling what I'm told is the "inevitable" surgery date. My choices are dire: Either I'm laden with pills for this and that or they want to cut me up, chop it off, or stick in some mechanical doodad. So went the too, too familiar orthopedic visit when I asked if there were any new techniques or options for healing my aching shoulder. I'm a layman so I didn't know a rotator cuff from my tibia tuberosity. All that I knew is that I had lost full range of motion, as was said and jotted down in my file. I could ice it, heat it, numb it out, x-ray it, MRI it...but I knew in the doc's mind that it would just be more pills or another surgery. Or as my doc actually said, "It's age, learn to live with it." Which I did for five years!

Then while having a wonderful massage, Peggy says that she has a way to ease my pain. From a massage therapist? But then she starts working on muscles and tendons and pressing on this and that, working parts of me no doctor's ever said was a pathway to healing. Sure, she's giving me a Latin name for this and that and honestly I'm getting a bit unsettled with this very unusual approach but when she asks me to raise my arm and move it this way and that way, believe me, within twenty minutes she had me thinking that the ole hook shot was back. Months later, I am still walking around with full range of movement, no pills, no schedule for surgery, and a lot of trust in what a massage therapist can do for my rotator cuff injury. Of course I did my "homework" – all the suggestions in her Ouch to Aaah Self-Care book. Listening to Peggy and/or working with a massage therapist whom she has trained is, quite simply, a slam-dunk!" (Frank Kroncke, Wisconsin)

"Peggy was a miracle worker in my life. A number of years ago I started hurting on the outside of the upper part of my right arm. I couldn't sleep on my stomach or that side a because of the extreme pain. Eventually, the same thing happened on the left arm. At this point I went to my physician who gave me some kind of medication which didn't help. Then he sent me to a specialist who gave me a different medication which didn't help. Then the specialist sent me to physical therapy. I got worse. After about eight weeks of physical therapy, the specialist decided I would need surgery. I walked out of his office and thought I am worse off than when I started this, I'll just live with it.

About that time a friend in Dallas who goes to a massage therapist told her about me. She asked a simple question which neither doctor had asked me, "Does it hurt all of the time or just when she raises her hands or pushes her arms back." That was easy, I could work with my hands in front of me with no pain. That massage therapist referred me to Peggy. At my first appointment she told me she that I had rotator cuff problems. I was very skeptical. Her manipulation seemed very minor to me, and she gave me instructions for a simple exercise. I believe it was after the second visit that I raised my arms up and then up and up and I was free of pain. This was almost unbelievable. I will be eternally grateful for Peggy. The medical profession misdiagnosed me and was about to do surgery on me. It scares me every time I think about it. Now, every time I think of Peggy Lamb, I thank God for her. Her caring concern and her expertise cured me of rotator cuff problems."
(Dr. Beverly Chiodo, Texas)

Ninety percent of all rotator cuff injuries arise from **poor posture and incorrect shoulder mechanics** which in turn cause:

■   Strength imbalance between the muscles that roll the shoulder forward and back (internal and external rotators). The internal rotators of the shoulder joint (humerus bone) outnumber the external rotators. What do people do when they go to the gym? Strength train the internal rotators such as the mighty pectoralis major and ignore the external rotators! I'll cover this in more depth in the section entitled *"A Lesson in Shoulder Mechanics"*.

■   Inflamed and possibly fibrotic rotator cuff muscles and tendons and trigger points in the muscles which interfere with the ability of the cuff to function properly.

■   Weak scapulae stabilizers (the muscles that anchor the shoulder blades).

■   Weak and overstretched scapulae retractors (the muscles that pull the shoulder blades together - rhomboids and middle traps).

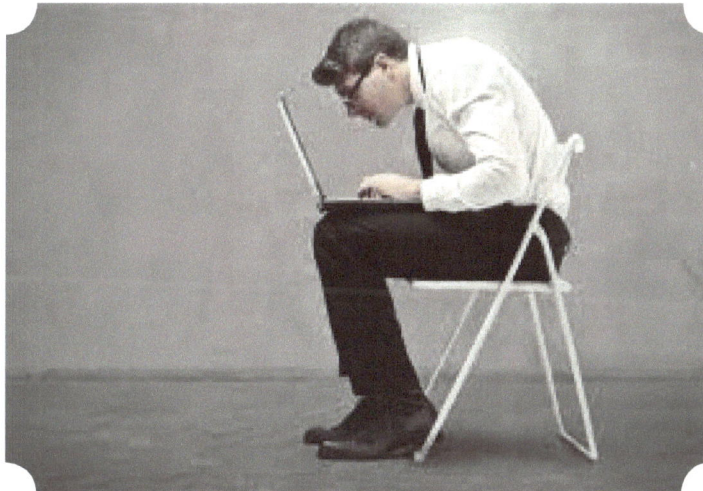

Rotator Cuff Muscles

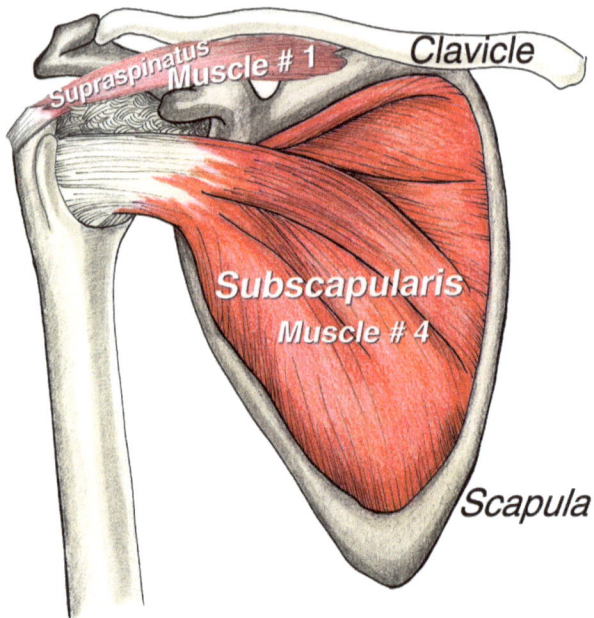

Front view of the rotator cuff muscles

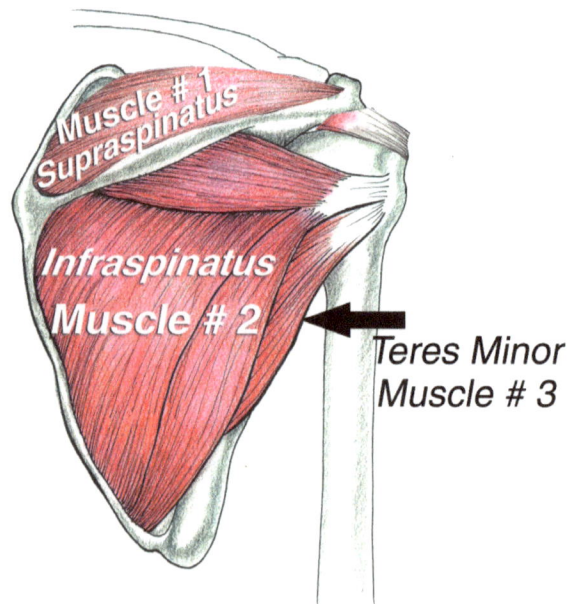

Back view of the rotator cuff muscles

A vitally important concept in this book is that of *referred pain from trigger points.* A trigger point is a hyper-irritable point in a muscle that refers or radiates pain to another part of the body. Let's look at the trigger point referral patterns for the rotator cuff muscles.

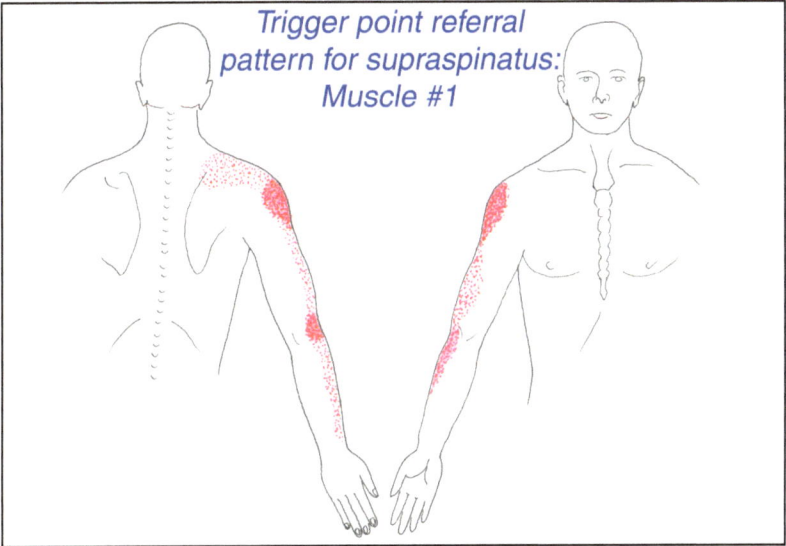

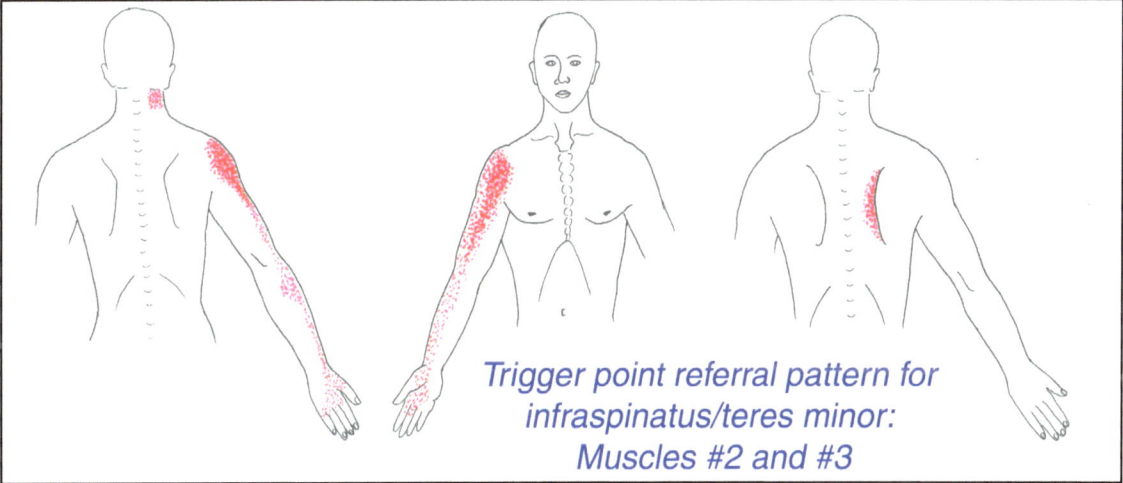

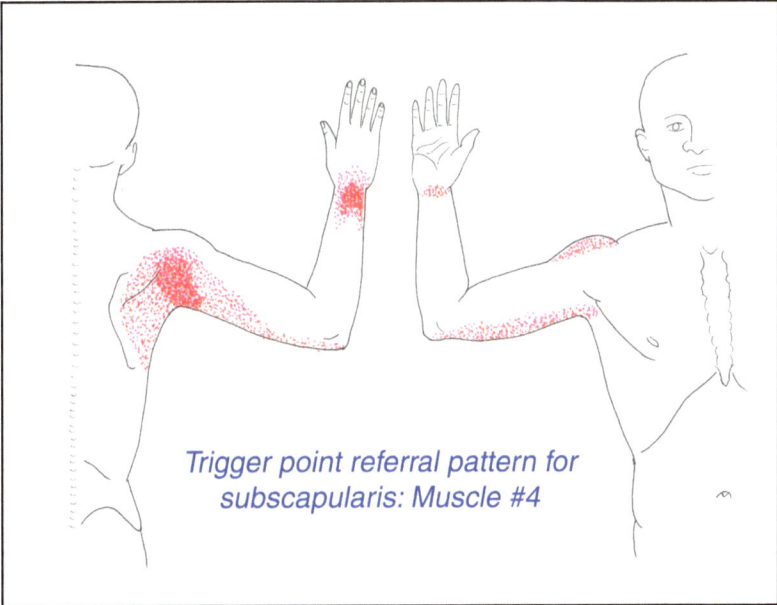

Trigger point referral pattern for supraspinatus: Muscle #1

Trigger point referral pattern for infraspinatus/teres minor: Muscles #2 and #3

Trigger point referral pattern for subscapularis: Muscle #4

DO YOU RECOGNIZE ANY OF YOUR PAIN PATTERNS?

As you can see, these trigger points are responsible for much of the shoulder pain people suffer. My clients have been amazed when I show them these trigger point patterns. If they've seen a doctor, they usually exclaim, "How come my doctor never showed me this?" I gently explain that many doctors are not educated about trigger points. Ironically, two pioneers in trigger point research were Drs. Janet Travell and David Simons, both MD's. Dr. Janet Travell was the White House physician during the Kennedy and Johnson administrations. She helped John F. Kennedy so much with his back pain from injuries he sustained during World War II with procaine injections into trigger points that he made her the White House physician.

Most of the time these trigger points are caused by poor posture and incorrect shoulder mechanics. The trigger point can feel like a small pea buried deep in the muscle. These hyper-irritable points place a constant strain on the muscle, restricting circulation and producing noxious chemical by-products. The resulting deprivation of oxygen and nutrients can perpetuate trigger points for years. *Conventional pain treatment often fails because it focuses on the pain and not the cause of the pain.*

ROTATOR CUFF INJURIES CAN INCLUDE ALL OR SOME OF THE FOLLOWING:

- Tears in muscles and/or tendons.

- Tendonitis or tendonosis (breakdown of collagen fibers) in tendons.

- Trigger points in muscles.

- Adaptive shortening of internal rotators of the shoulder joint (humerus). This shortening of the internal rotators pulls the head of the humerus (the big ball on top of your upper arm) forward, creating a painful over-stretched state of muscles # 3 and 4 (infraspinatus and teres minor).

- Impingement of bursa and tendons.

- Formation of scar tissue (adhesions) that decrease the muscle's ability to contract and stretch. Scar tissue often binds together damaged and undamaged tissue resulting in adhesions, causing pain, re-injury, and restricted range of movement. Scar tissue primarily forms in ligaments, muscles, tendons, fascia, and joint capsules.

- Injury such as a fall onto the shoulder.

- Bicipital tendonitis (inflammation of the long head of the biceps) which sometimes accompanies rotator cuff injuries.

The Rotator Cuff

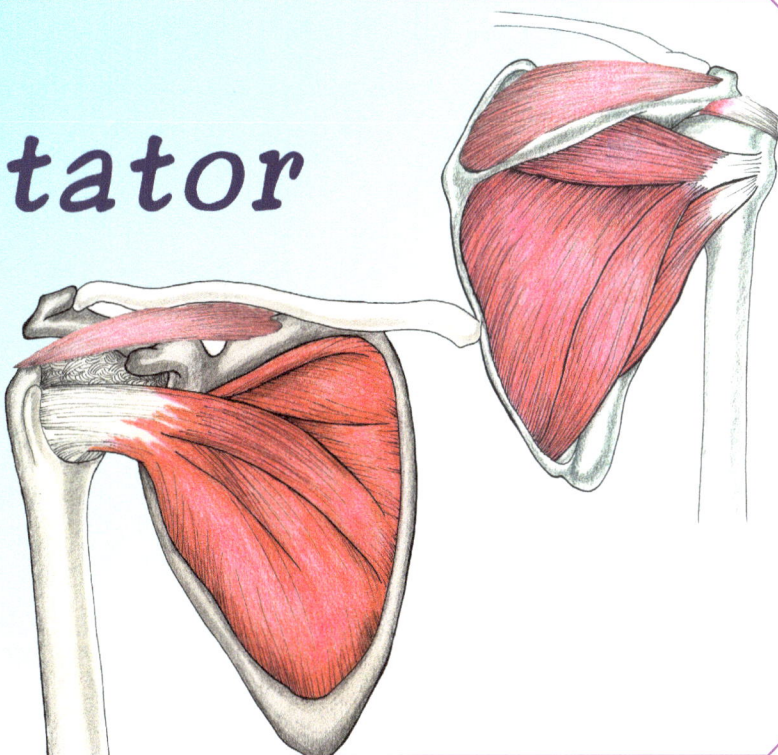

THE ROTATOR CUFF

All shoulder pain involves the rotator cuff to some degree. It is the commander and chief of the shoulder complex. Let's start by understanding the rotator cuff.

The rotator cuff is a combination of four muscles:

•*Supraspinatus (Muscle #1)*
•*Infraspinatus (Muscle #2)*
•*Teres minor (Muscle #3)*
•*Subscapularis; (Muscle #4)*

Together they are commonly known as the "SITS" muscles. They work together to stabilize the head of the humerus during all shoulder movements (essentially most upper body movements).

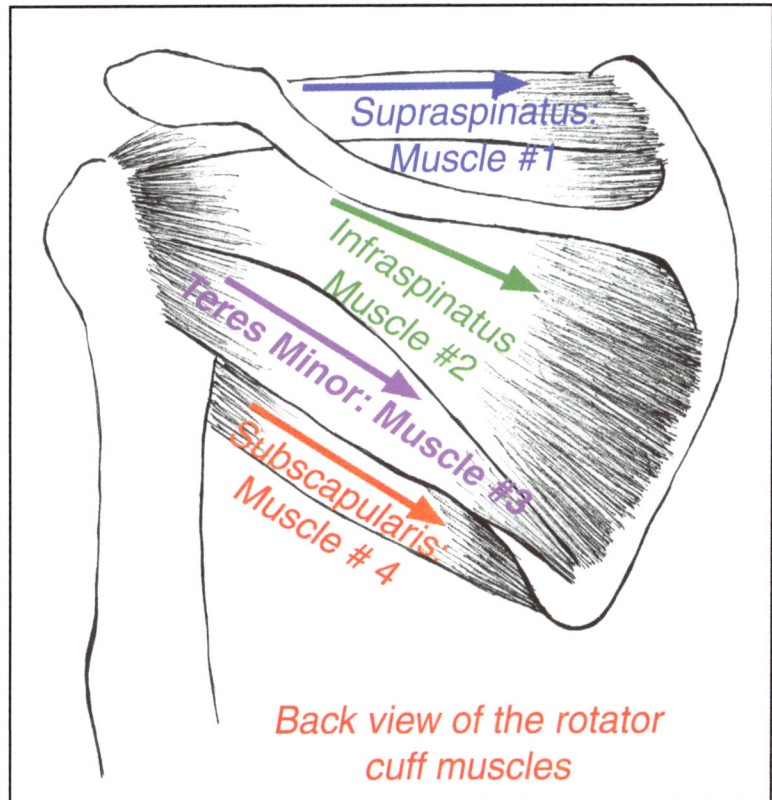

Supraspinatus: Muscle #1

Infraspinatus Muscle #2

Teres Minor: Muscle #3

Subscapularis: Muscle # 4

Back view of the rotator cuff muscles

"SITS" keeps the humerus stable and centered in the shoulder joint. Think of them as guy wires pulling on a tent pole.

•**Muscle #1** (supraspinatus) pulls the head of the humerus into the shoulder joint from above.
•**Muscle #2** (infraspinatus) pulls it in from the rear.
•**Muscle #3** (teres minor) pulls it in from bottom/rear.
•**Muscle #4** (subscapularis) pulls it in from the bottom/front *(see graphic above)*.

Some sources define the cuff as the tendons of these four muscles but we will use a broader definition that includes the muscles.

A healthy rotator cuff stabilizes the shoulder joint so we can swim, dance, play tennis, throw a ball, play golf; etc. An injured cuff compromises the function of all the muscles surrounding the joint.

Another way the rotator cuff works is as a decelerator or braking system to slow things down. If you throw a ball or swing a tennis racket, first you externally rotate your shoulder as a wind up; then forcefully internally rotate as you throw or hit the ball as shown in the picture to your right. What keeps your arm from flying off your body? The rotator cuff, specifically the infraspinatus and teres minor. These two small powerhouses are the only external rotators of the shoulder joint. They have to work very hard to counterbalance the powerful internal rotators which outnumber them.

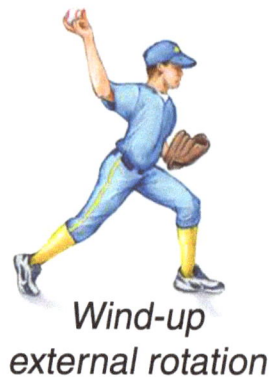

Throwing the ball internal rotation

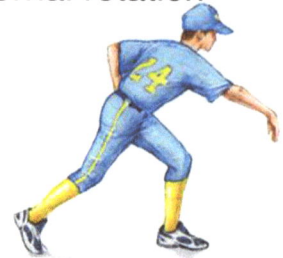

Wind-up external rotation

In addition to the stabilizing and deceleration functions, the rotator cuff has another big job. It performs movements*: *(these terms defined in next chapter)*

     1. Subscapularis: internal rotation
     2. Infraspinatus and teres minor: external rotation of the humerus
     3. Supraspinatus: abduction of the humerus

In summary, the rotator cuff:

1. Stabilizes the head of the humerus during all shoulder joint movements.
2. Decelerates the arm when you throw something or swing a golf club, etc.
3. Provides movement: internal/external rotation and abduction of the humerus.

These are busy muscles that are constantly multitasking!

A Lesson in Shoulder Mechanics

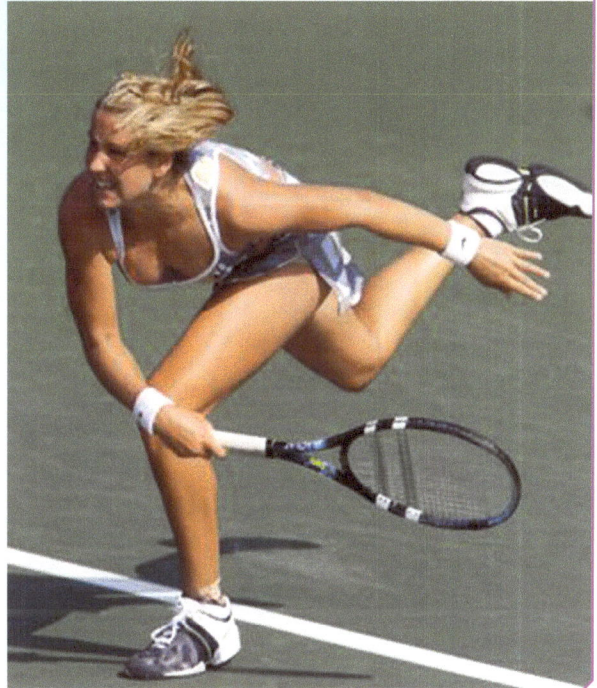

A Lesson In Shoulder Mechanics

Now it's time for you to learn a little about your own anatomy. Don't be scared - you won't be tested and you will benefit so much by knowing yourself a little better. Our goal here is to help you recognize your habitual patterns of movement and correct those that need change. This is a profoundly important step in your healing process and a way to prevent future problems with your shoulders. Let's start with the bones.

THE SHOULDER GIRDLE AND SHOULDER JOINT

The shoulder girdle consists of the scapulae (shoulder blades) and clavicles (collarbones). The shoulder joint is where the head of the humerus fits into the a socket (the glenoid fossa) created by the shoulder girdle.

BONES OF THE SHOULDER GIRDLE AND JOINT

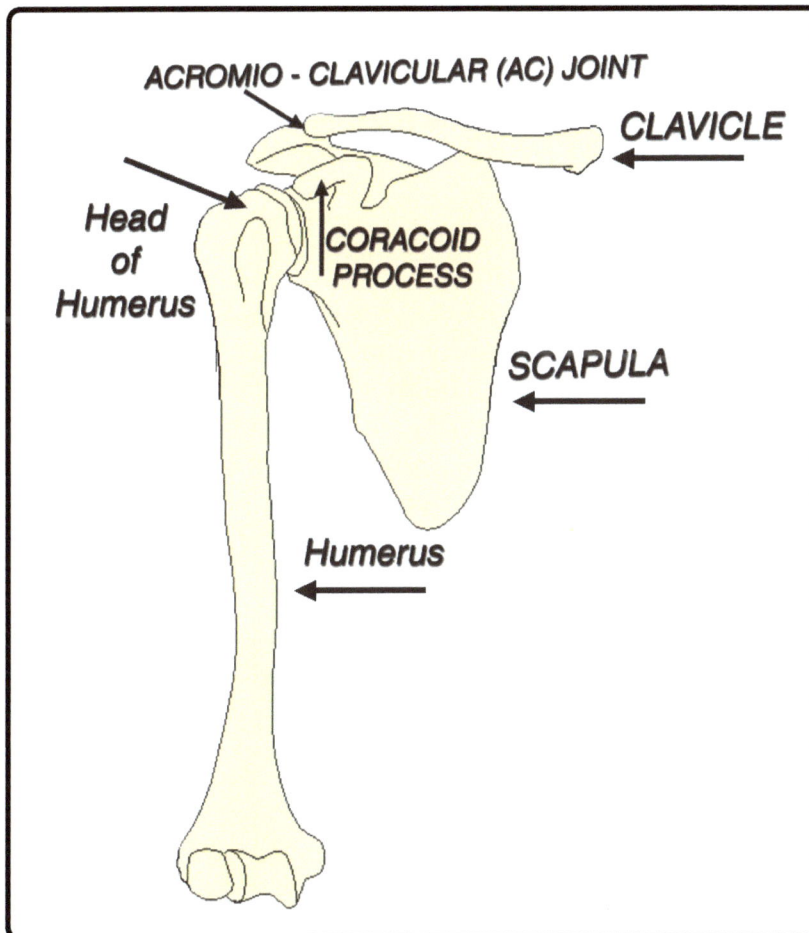

ACROMIO - CLAVICULAR (AC) JOINT

CLAVICLE

Head of Humerus

CORACOID PROCESS

SCAPULA

Humerus

FRONT VIEW

Movements of the shoulder joint: abduction, adduction, external rotation, internal rotation, flexion, extension, circumduction.

Not to worry - you don't have to memorize all of these. There are some that are quite important to know:

- **Abduction** of the shoulder joint (moving the arms away from the side of the body)
- **Adduction** of the shoulder joint (moving the arms back to the side of the body)
- **Internal rotation** of the shoulder joint (rolling the shoulder forward)
- **External rotation** of the shoulder joint (rolling the shoulder backward)

This happy fellow's arms are **ABDUCTED** or lifted away from the side of the body. When he brings his arms back to his sides, he's **ADDUCTING** his arms.

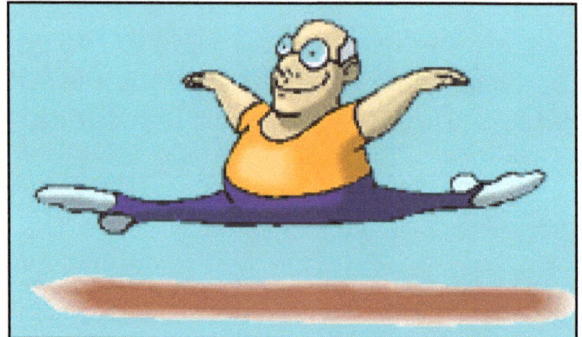

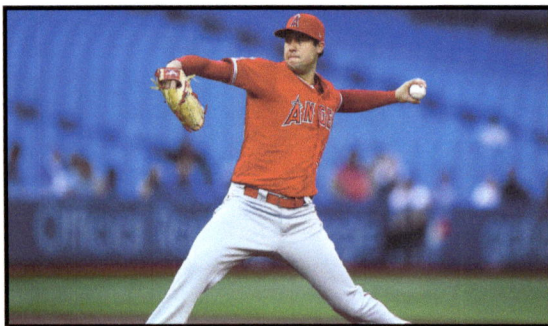

This baseball player's right shoulder is **INTERNALLY ROTATED.** Try this on your body:

Place your hand on the top of your shoulder. Feel for the big ball-like structure - that's the head of your humerus. Roll it forward. You've just internally rotated your shoulder joint. Do you spend most of your time with your shoulders internally rotated? If so, you can start right now to change that! You'll find out soon why it's not the optimum position for your shoulder joint.

This javelin thrower's right shoulder is **EXTERNALLY ROTATED.** Try this on your body:

Find the head of your humerus again. This time roll it backward. You've just externally rotated your shoulder joint.
Neutral shoulder is somewhere between internal and external rotation. Can you find that on yourself? It's the position we want to spend most of our time in.

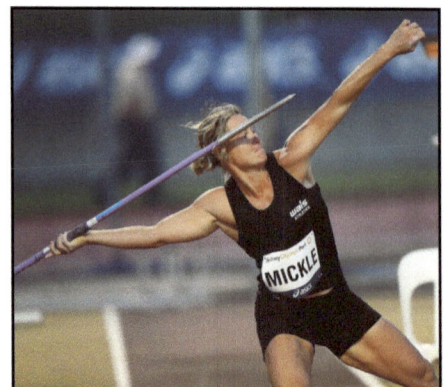

Movements of the shoulder girdle (*shoulder blades and collarbones*): elevation, depression, retraction, protraction, upward and downward rotation.

Again - you don't have to memorize all of these. The important ones are:

•**Retraction** of the shoulder blades (squeezing the shoulder blades together)
•**Protraction** of the shoulder blades (moving the shoulder blades away from each other)
•**Elevation** of the shoulder blades (lifting the shoulder blades up)
•**Depression** of the shoulder blades (dropping the shoulder blades down)

Squeezing the shoulder blades together is **Retraction** of the shoulder girdle (scapula/collarbones). In the picture to your right, can you see how her shoulder blades are coming toward each other? Try it on yourself: Imagine there's a lemon between your shoulder blades and squeeze that lemon!

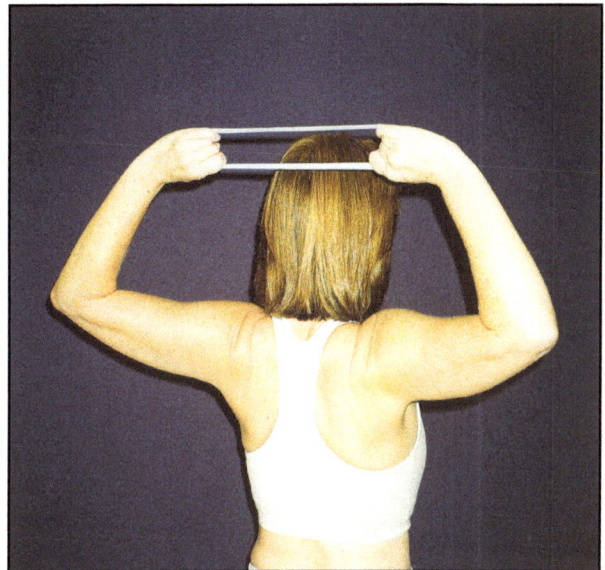

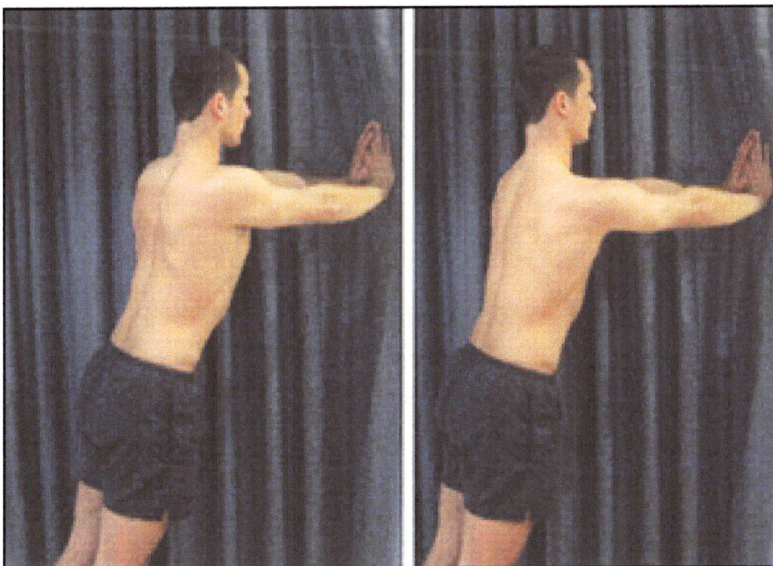

The opposite of **Retraction** is **Protraction** of the shoulder girdle (scapula/collarbones). In the picture on the left, his shoulder blades are squeezed together and in the picture on the right, his shoulder blades are coming apart in **Protraction.** Try it on yourself. Move your shoulder blades away from each other. Now, find a position for your shoulder blades that's somewhere in the middle. We'll call that position neutral shoulder blades and that's where we want our shoulder blades most of the time. Where are your shoulder blades most of the time?

16

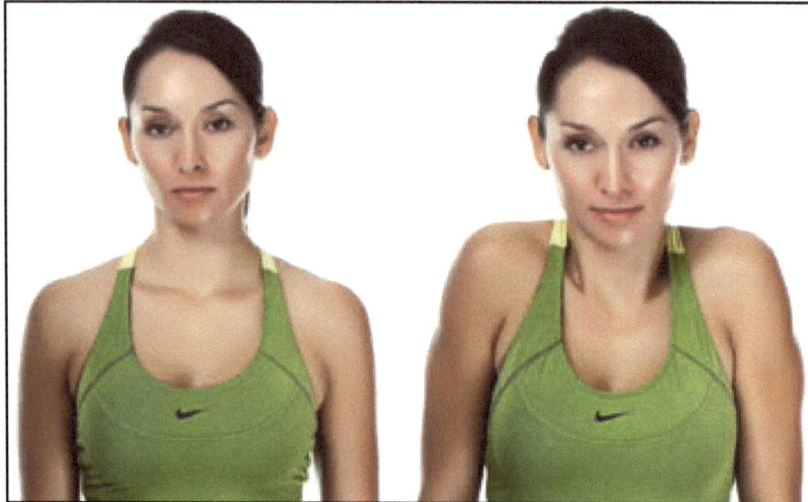

Last but not least is **ELEVATION** and **DEPRESSION** of the shoulder blades. Raise your shoulders towards your ears, then let them drop back down. Letting our shoulders rise toward the ears is a common response to tension and stress. Habitually holding them there impacts how effectively the rotator cuff can work. So, let those shoulders slide down. You don't want to end up like this poor gal, do you?

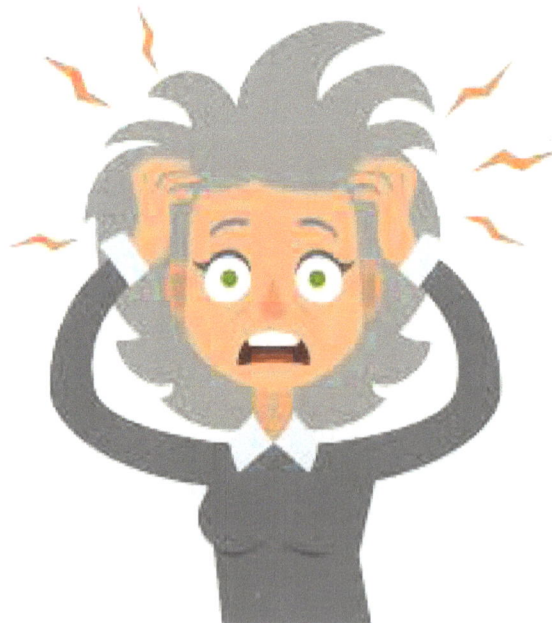

Our next quest is to delve a bit deeper into habitual habits of movement and posture. This is a fun, if a bit unorthodox, exercise to enlighten you about your habitual shoulder mechanics. In the process you'll learn a host of things, including the principles of proper shoulder mechanics.

ARE YOU A GREAT DANE OR A BULL DOG?

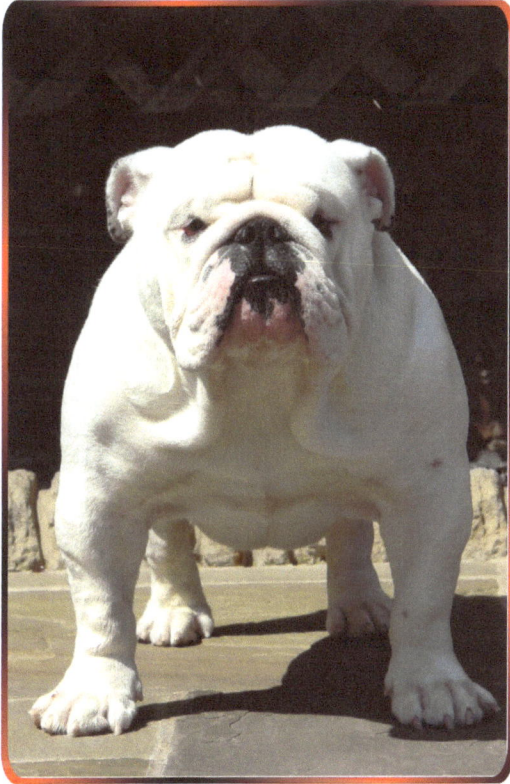

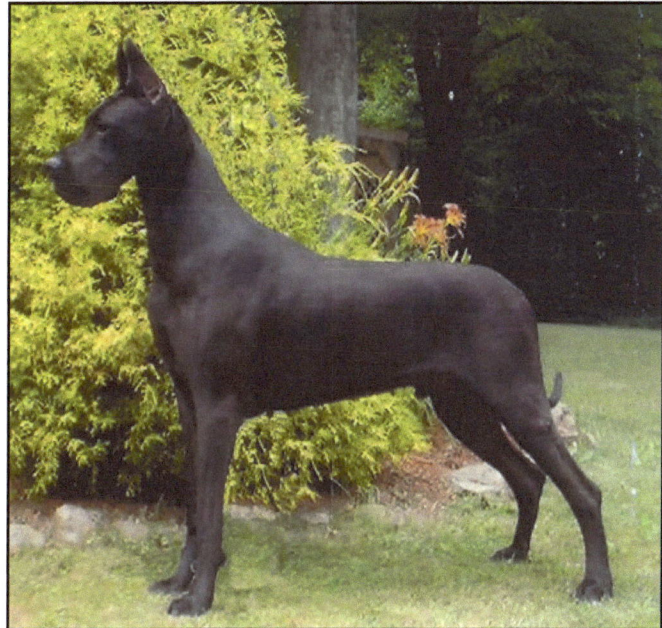

You 'll be getting down on your hands and knees (nothing kinky, I promise). Take this booklet with you, as I'll be posing four questions to you. Write the answers to your questions in the space provided. I suggest reading through the exercise before doing it. Once you're on your hands and knees, note your answers in your mind; then write them down when you are finished.

OK, ready? Get down on your hands and knees. Here's your four questions:

1. Notice if your elbows are straight or bent: _____

2. Notice if your shoulder joints (that's the head of your humerus, the big ball at the top of your upper arm) are internally (rolled forward) rotated or externally (rolled backward) rotated: _____

3. Are your shoulder blades coming toward each other or away from each other (retraction or protraction)? _____

4. Does it feel like the weight of your upper body is being transferred through the center of your joints?_____

Great! Remember to write your answers down so you have a record you can refer to. This will help you track your progress.

Let's analyze this information by comparing bull dogs and great danes.

BULL DOG

1. Bent elbows
2. Internally rotated shoulder joints
3. Shoulder blades going away from each other
4. Weight is being transferred in a zig-zag manner

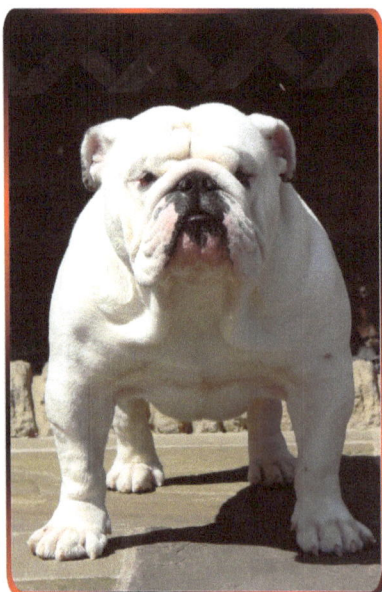

GREAT DANE

1. Straight elbows
2. Externally rotated shoulder joints
3. Shoulder blades going toward each other
4. Weight is being transferred through the center of the joints

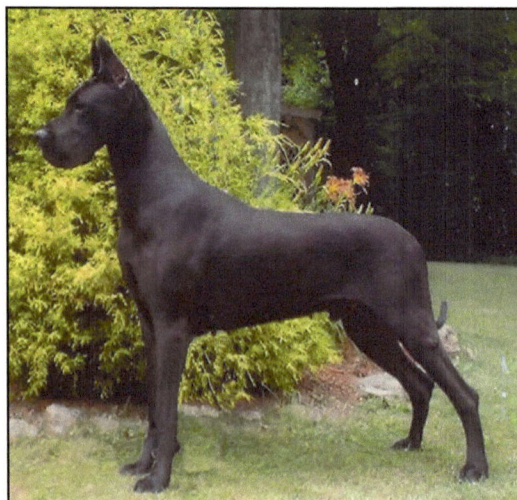

Which one are you - a bull dog or great dane? If you're a great dane, bully for you! If you're a bull dog, you've just learned and identified some habitual postural/movement patterns that need to be changed. Bully for you too because awareness is the first step toward change.

Why is it better to be a Great Dane than a Bull dog? Bull dog lovers, please forgive me! They are both great breeds. The four elements of a great dane -- *straight elbows, externally rotated shoulder joints, shoulder blades going toward each other and weight being transferred through the center of the joints* -- create a stable base for weight bearing. The picture below shows an example of correct hands and knees position. If you were a bull dog, I'm sure you could feel that the weight of your upper body was being transferred in a zig-zag manner. This means that your muscles, instead of your bones, were bearing weight, which is not in their job description. It is the job of our wonderfully strong bones to bear weight. The bent elbows, internally rotated shoulder joints, and shoulder blades going away from each other puts stress on some soft tissue structures that you'll learn about next.

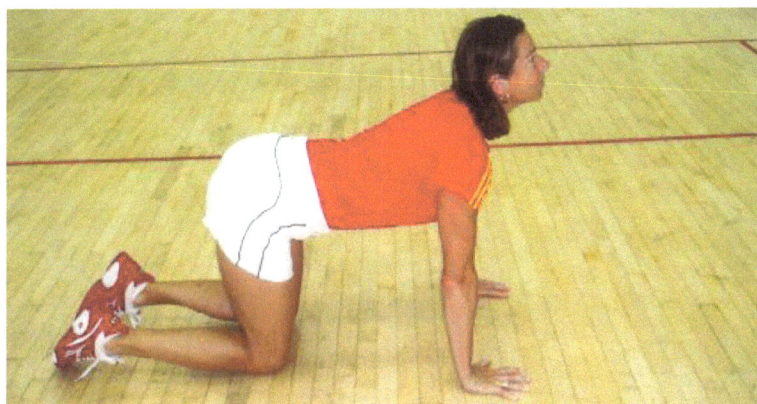

What about push-ups? When you do a push up you pass *through* a bull dog phase. It's ok to be a bull dog for short periods of time; just don't hang out there.

For you Yoga enthusiasts, this information has important relevance for a pose you do all the time: *Downward Facing Dog*. It was from years of incorrectly doing Down Dog that I injured my rotator cuff. In that pose and any other upper body weight-bearing pose, make sure you are a proud and strong Great Dane! An image I like to use to create my stable upper-body base is that there are eyes on the inside of my elbows. I rotate my elbows so that the "eyes" are looking at each other. This small movement lengthens the elbows and creates a strong external rotation in the shoulder joint.

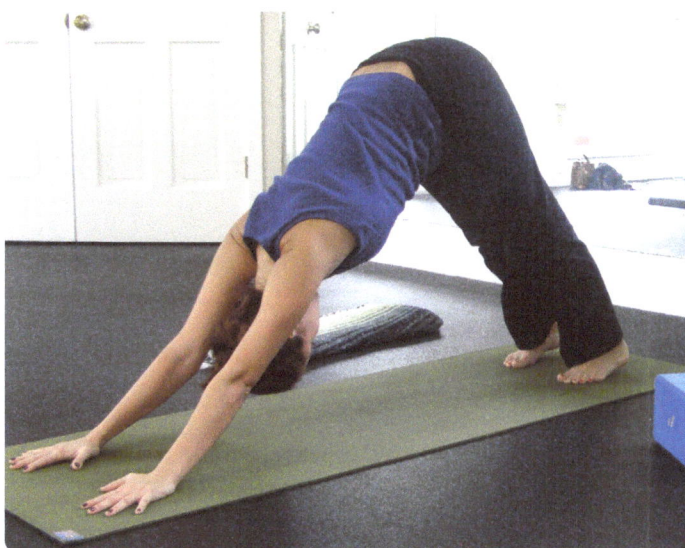

Here's another little test that can reveal important information about your habitual shoulder mechanics.

Imagine you are standing in your kitchen and your morning coffee is just about ready. You reach up for a coffee cup in a cabinet in front and above your head. How do you reach for that cup? Do you raise your arm straight up in front of you, as if you were High Fiveing a friend? Or do you take the long way by raising your arm away from your side, then crossing it over in front of your face? If you're a High Fiver, you get a High Five. If you like to take the long way, I want you to start High Fiveing to get your coffee cup and anything else you reach for. Why? Read on.

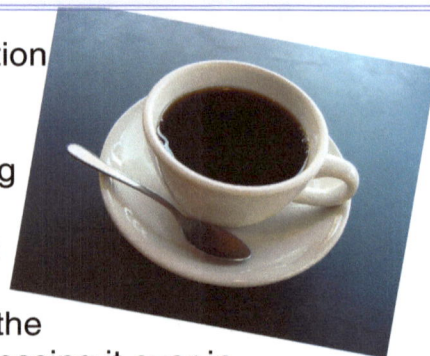

What I'm illustrating are the dangers of a posture with habitually internally rotated shoulder joints (remember, that's where the big ball-like structure in the upper arms connects to the torso). This puts a quite a strain on the muscles that internally rotate the shoulder and the muscles that externally rotate the shoulder. The internal rotators become locked-short (frozen in a shortened position) while the external rotators become locked-long or over-stretched (frozen in a stretched position). This causes a strength imbalance that affects the rotator cuff's ability to function effectively As, I've said, most of the clients I've seen over the years with shoulder pain are paying the price for this kind of posture.

To add fuel to the fire, when you raise your arm away from your side (abduction), with your shoulder joint rolled forward (internal rotation), there are a number of structures that get impinged and compressed. This impingement/ compression causes micro-tearing in these structures. Over time these micro-tears become larger and begin reporting pain and/or loss of range of motion. This is why shoulder pain usually makes itself known in middle age.

ALWAYS ABDUCT WITH THE THUMB UP!

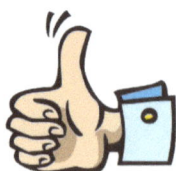

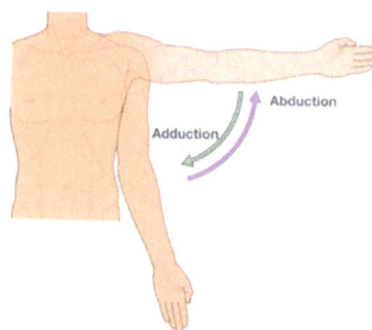

Abduction

Adduction

Greater
Tubercle

Lesser
Tubercle

Figure C

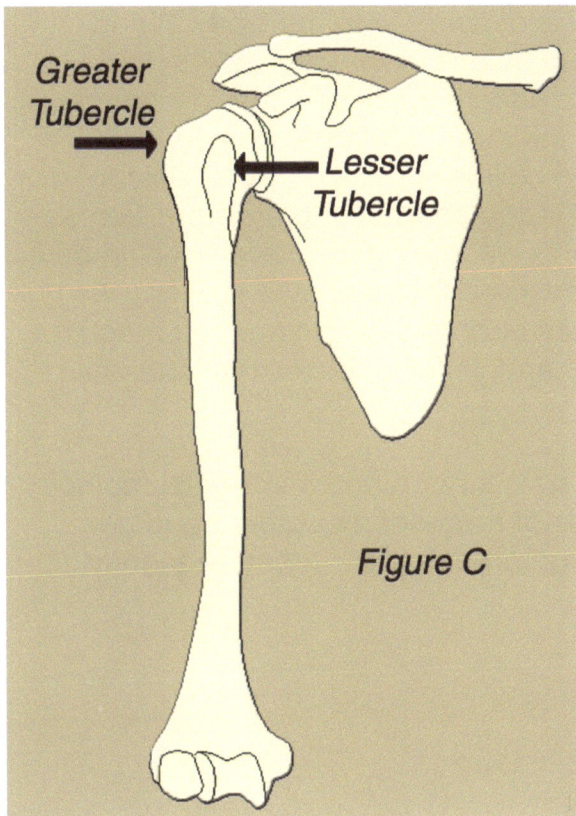

Now let's consider that nasty and pervasive habit of letting the shoulders roll forward into internal rotation in a little more detail with interactive anatomy. Look at **Figure C** on the left. There are two bony landmarks labeled the greater tubercle and the lesser tubercle. Find the greater tubercle on yourself.

Place your hand on the very top your upper arm. It's a rather bumpy place. Staying on the humerus bone, feel around for big bumps. You want the one that's on the back portion of the humerus. There's a number of bumps, so if you get lost, not to worry - this exploration will still work. Once you're in the general vicinity of this big bump called the greater tubercle, roll the humerus forward, like you did before in internal rotation. What happens to the greater tubercle? It goes along for the ride, right?

Excellent, you did great!

With your shoulder rolled forward and keeping your fingers glued to the big bump, lift your arm away from your side. Lift it as high as you can. At a certain point, you should feel a restriction of movement. That restriction is the greater tubercle colliding (**ouch!**) with a part of the shoulder blade known as the acromion process. Victims of this collision are several key structures of the shoulder joint:

1. Supraspinatus (Muscle #1) tendon.
2. Sub-acromial bursa (yes, this is why so many people are diagnosed with shoulder bursitis. Usually the doctor prescribes an anti-inflammatory without looking into the root causes of the bursitis).
3. Long head of the biceps.

In fact, this superior aspect of the shoulder joint is called the *impingement area*.

The graphic below is a good illustration of what actually happens when we roll the shoulder forward in internal rotation and lift the arm away from the body. When the humerus is internally rotated, the greater tubercle rolls forward, taking that supraspinatus (Muscle #1) tendon along for the ride. In the graphic below the greater tubercle is covered by muscles. Since the supraspinatus (Muscle #1) attaches to the top of the greater tubercle, it will collide with a bony process on your shoulder blade when the humerus is abducted in the internally rotated position as shown in **Figure D.** Just imagine how many times people do this on any given day! Remember the coffee cup exercise? If you discovered that you take the long way to get your cup, micro-tearing of these structures happens each time you reach for that cup. Eventually these structures get fed up and yell a loud and unmistakable *"OUCH!"*

The sub-acromial bursa lives on top of Muscle #1's tendon and it too gets impinged and compressed, resulting in inflammation, loss of range of movement and pain. On the next page you'll see a graphic of the structures that are most frequently torn and damaged.

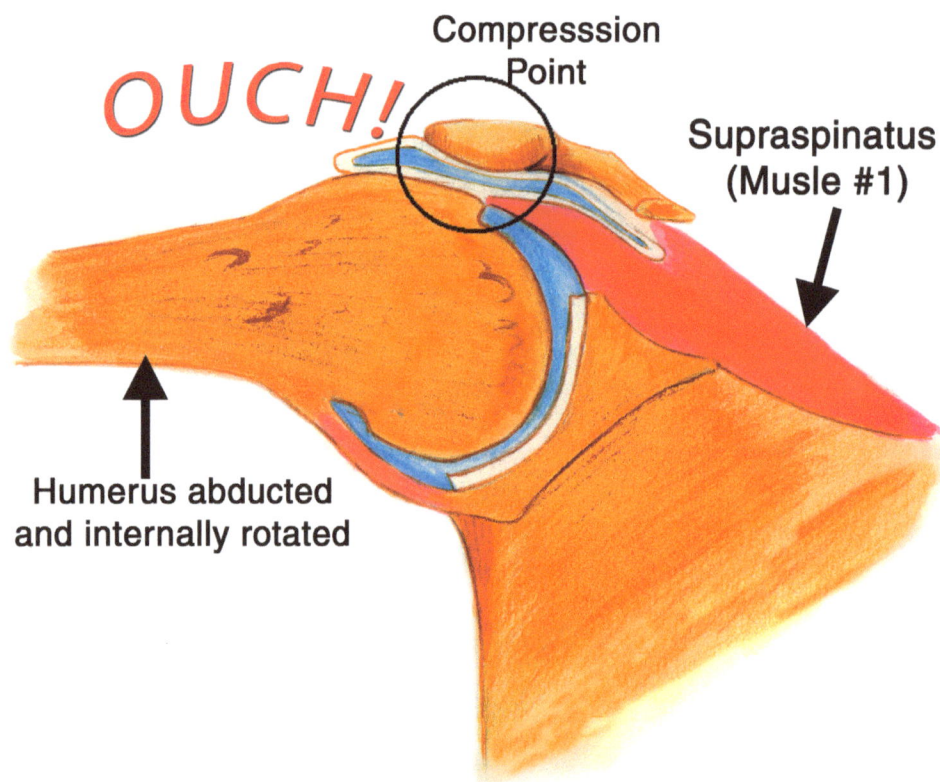

Figure D

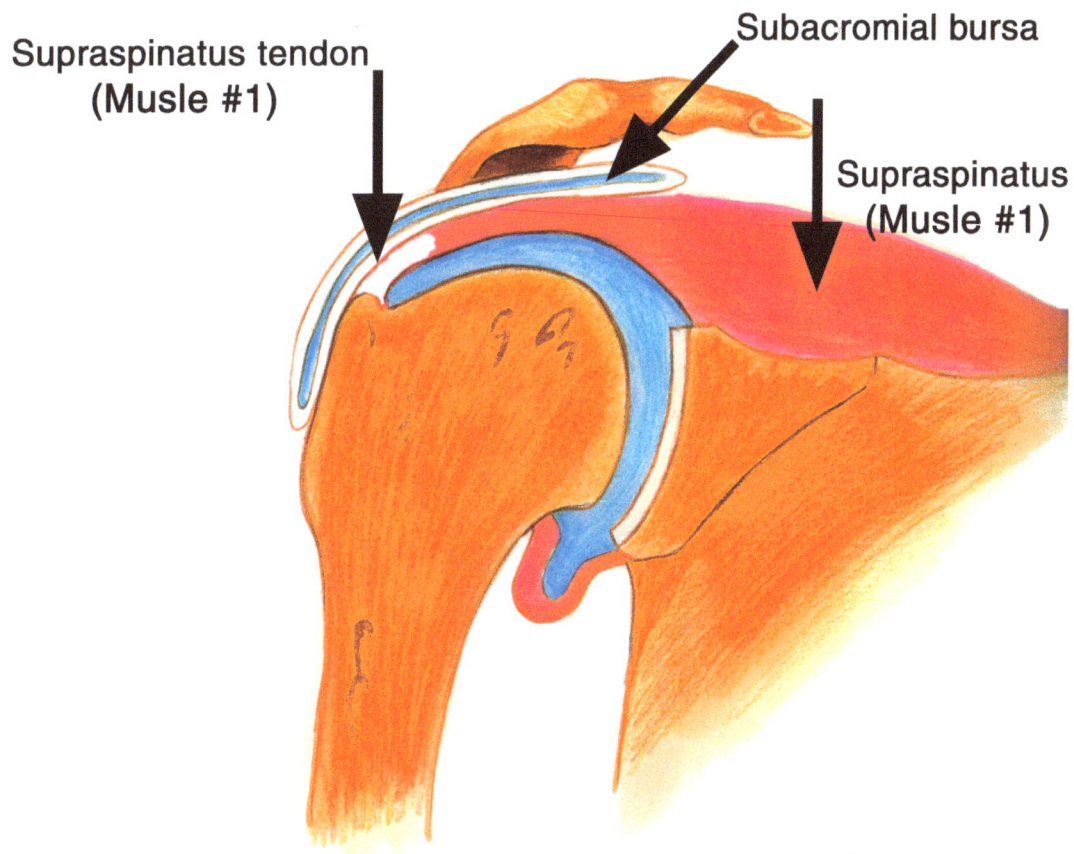

**Supraspinatus tendon
(Musle #1)**

Subacromial bursa

**Supraspinatus
(Musle #1)**

Figure E

Figure E shows the humerus in a neutral position. Some bones and bony prominences have been removed to better show the structures of the supraspinatus muscle and tendon (Muscle #1), and the subacromial bursa. These structures, along with the long head of the biceps(shown on next page) are in the impingement zone and are frequent guilty culprits in shoulder problems.

The supraspinatus (Muscle #1) muscle/tendon unit is the most frequently torn rotator cuff muscle. Most rotator cuff surgeries are performed to re-attach a torn supraspinatus as shown in **Figure F**.

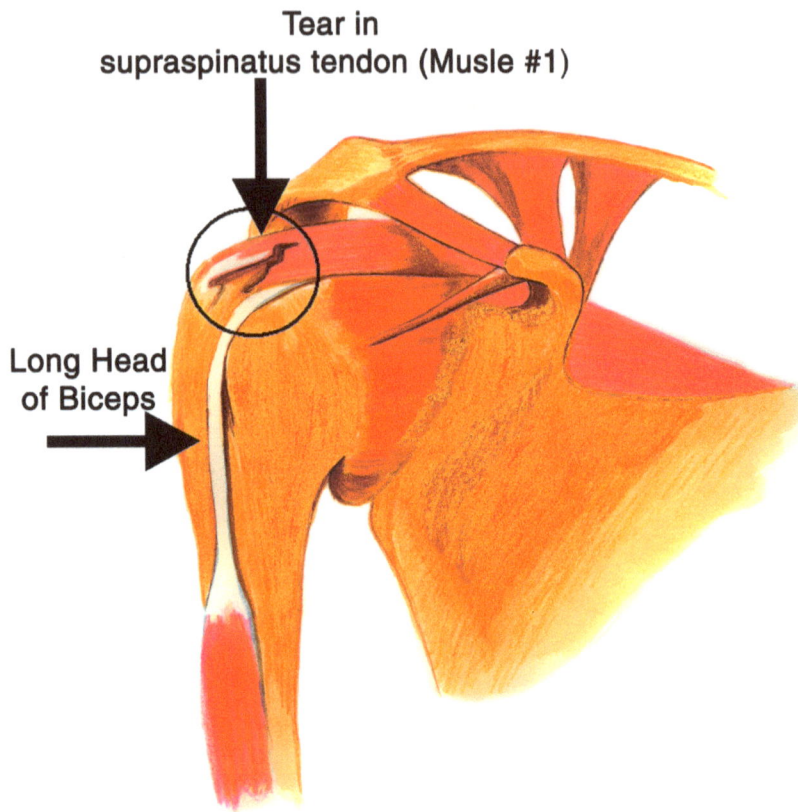

Tear in
supraspinatus tendon (Musle #1)

Long Head
of Biceps

Figure F

Internal rotation is our friend! It allows us to do many movements. But it is not a friendly position to call "home." Home position for bones should be in neutral. In neutral, our wonderful bones can be the weight supporting structures they were designed for and transfer weight through the center of the joints. With our bones centered in their proper homes, our muscles can cease to be weight supporting structures, giving them the freedom to move our bones and allowing us to move with greater ease and vitality and to express ourselves through our bodies.

Stretches
Strength
Training
and more

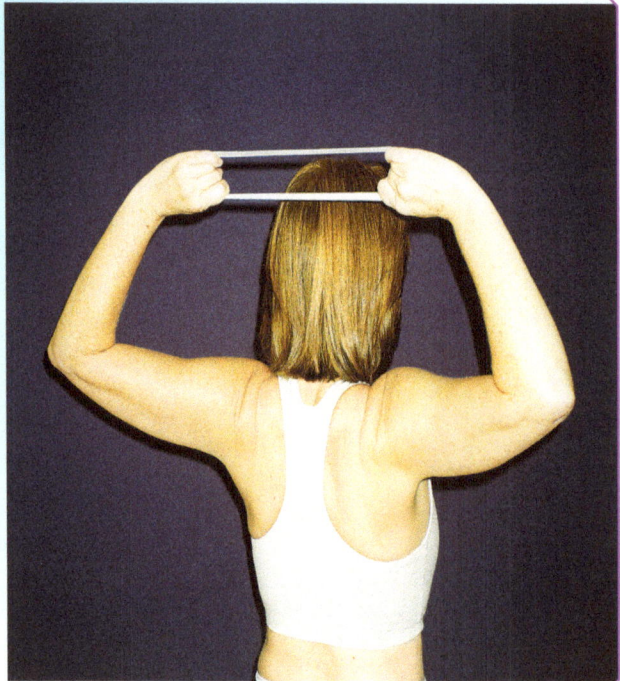

A Word of Advice

Your sleep position, stretches and strength training are essential ingredients for your recovery. This means that you have to do them! You will get out of this program what you put in. Inspire yourself to create and stick to a daily routine. If you're a golfer, visualize swinging your golf club freely and fluidly with no pain. Or visualize putting on your clothes with no pain and grinning from ear to ear with the a new-found sense of pain-free movement. See yourself with full range of movement in your shoulders, arms held high, saying an emphatic "YES" to your recovery. Visualization is a proven strategy for creating efficient and functional neuro-muscular pathways.

Approach the stretches and strength training with a gentle attitude. Rotator cuff injuries can take a long time to heal; allow the natural organic healing process to occur. Pushing from a place of impatience and frustration is understandable but counter-productive. Even if no results are discernible; healing **is** taking place - if you're doing your part. I remember the day I could fasten my seat belt with no pain. I didn't even notice at first. I had backed out of my driveway and was approaching the stop sign at the end of my block before the realization hit me. In stunned amazement, I pulled over, unfastened my seat belt with no pain and re-fastened it with no pain. That was about a year after my initial injury. The same will happen for you. One day you'll be able to move your arm with no pain. *Follow the way of nature; her secret is patience.*

At the end of the stretching and strength training sections, there are suggested daily routines of different levels. As your range of motion increases and your pain decreases, you can move to the next level. If your condition worsens, go back a level. Injury rehabilitation comes in waves - two steps forward, one step back. Expect that. On days when you're frustrated, impatient and angry, take some ice cubes outside and throw them with your good arm. It's quite therapeutic!

Your mantra: Strengthen what is weak, stretch what is short.

Sleep Positioning

One of the most important things you can do to help heal your shoulder is to make certain you are sleeping in the correct position. You will re-injure or aggravate a shoulder injury by improper sleep positioning. My injury took a quantum leap forward into healing when I changed my sleep position. It usually takes several months to change and integrate a new position. Sleeping on the back is fine as long as you don't cross your arms over your face or allow the shoulders to rest on the pillow - the shoulders should rest on the bed. If you are a stomach sleeper, I realize how hard it is to change that habit but make a valiant effort. At the very least, allow your shoulders to rest on the bed and not the pillow. The goal is to keep the shoulder joint in **neutral** as much as possible while you sleep.

Since most people are side-sleepers, photos A and B below show correct and incorrect side-lying sleep positions.

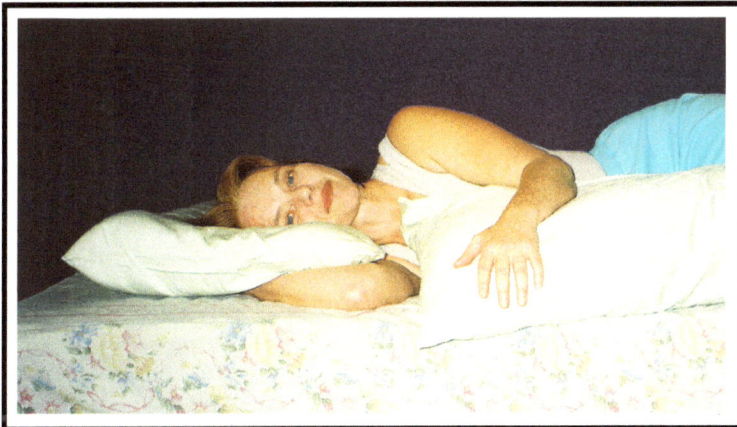

A. Correct use of a pillow to prevent shortening of the right subscapularis muscle (Muscle #4) and over-stretching of the left infraspinatus and teres minor muscles (Muscles # 2 and 3): The top arm is resting in a neutral position on the pillow. The lower arm in L shape under the pillow

B. Incorrect use of a pillow: this position shortens the right subscapularis muscle, (Muscle #4), (lower arm is held in an internally rotated position) and places the left (upper arm) infraspinatus and teres minor muscles (Muscles # 2 and 3) in a pain producing stretch.

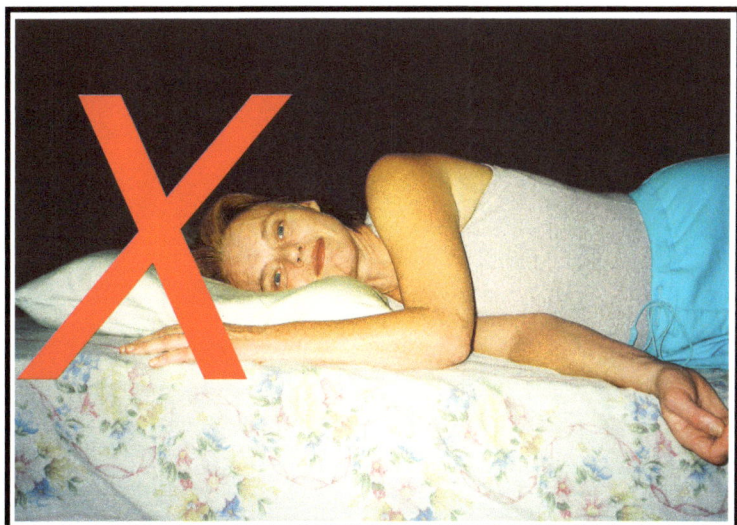

28

Simple Suggestions

1. Lie face-up on the floor with the arms in a **"T"** position at least once a day. This encourages the opening of the chest and external rotation of the shoulder joints with the body being supported by the floor and not weight bearing. To intensify this, a pillow can be placed either vertically along the spine or horizontally across the spine at the level of the lower edge of the shoulder blades. If necessary, bend knees and place feet flat on the floor to reduce lower back strain. Spend at least ten minutes in this position.

2. Swimming the back stroke is an excellent rehabilitation exercise for rotator cuffs. Even if you are not a swimmer, do the backstroke in a standing position within whatever movement range is comfortable. Again, this encourages external rotation of the shoulder joint.

3. If you are wearing belted pants, slip your thumbs through the belt loops on the sides of your hips. This places the shoulders in a neutral position.

4. When carrying heavy objects, keep the elbows close to the side.

5 Always raise your arm away from your side with your thumb up.

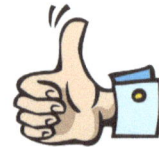

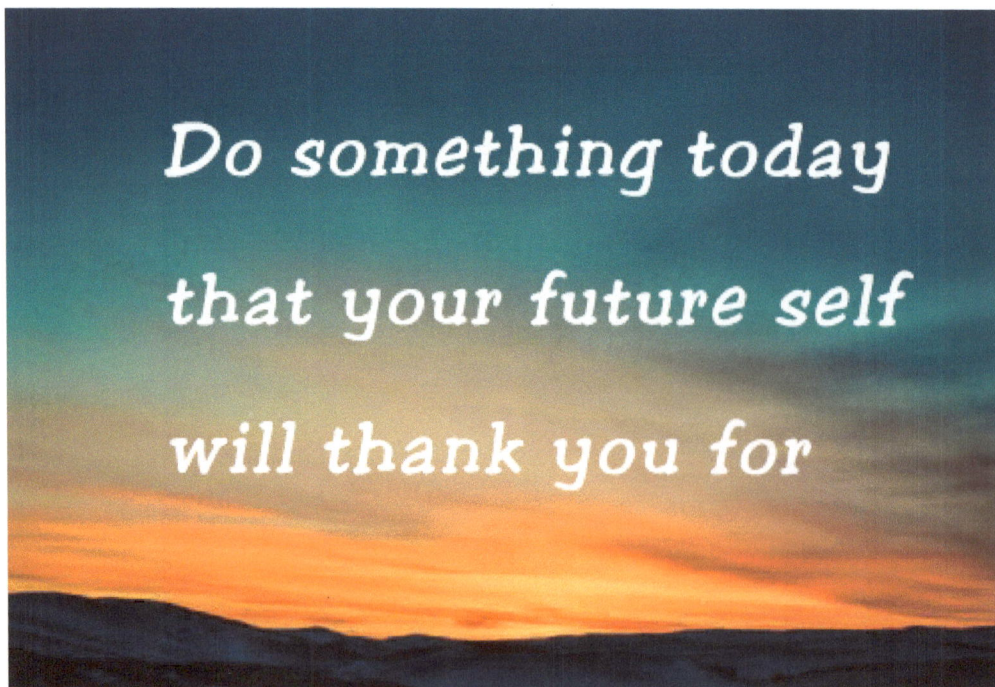

Do something today

that your future self

will thank you for

PENDULUM EXERCISE

PENDULUM EXERCISE: An excellent, gentle, releasing exercise for the shoulder joint is to come into a lunge position and allow the affected arm to hang down toward the floor. Your arm is passive during this exercise. Slowly shift your weight forward and back and side to side which creates a swing in your arm. This tractions the head of the humerus which tends to get jammed up in the joint.

Do this as needed; twice a day for five minutes is great.

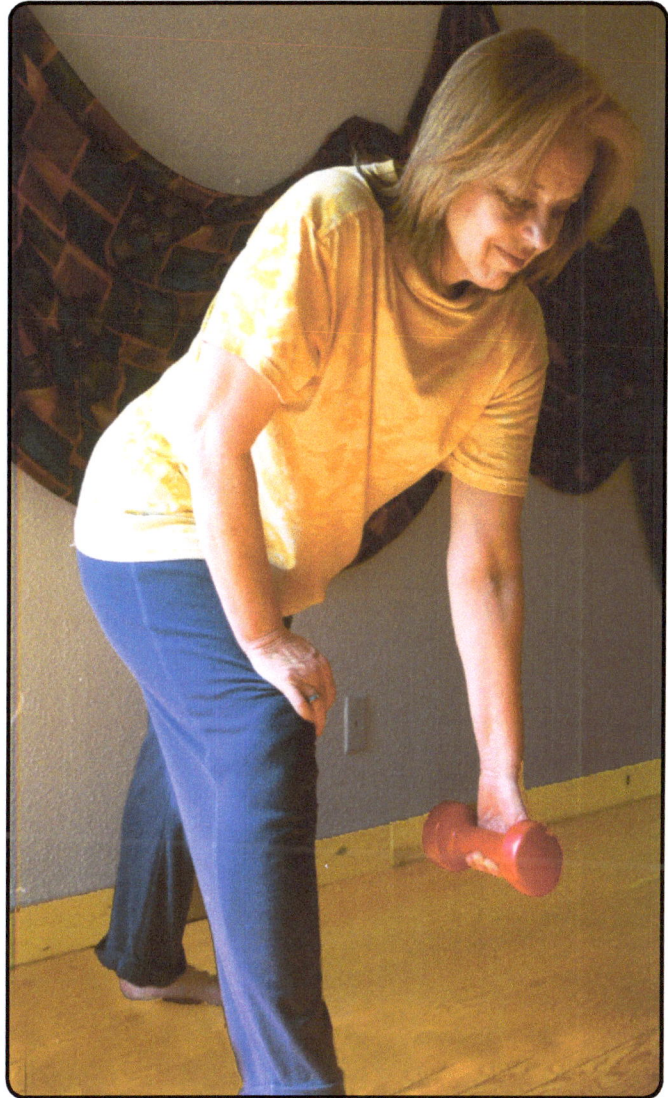

This section is divided into three categories:

- Humeral centration (a fancy word that means centering the head of the humerus in its socket)
- Stretches
- Stabilization exercises for the scapulae (shoulder blades)
- Strengthening of external rotators and scapulae retractors

This is an evergreen program; it won't go out of date. Yes, there are other exercises you can do but the ones in this book are the basics.

There are ten stretches: Commit to doing two a day
There are ten strengthening exercises: Commit to doing two a day
YOU CAN DO IT!!

Use sound judgment in making decisions about your ability to perform the exercises. Listen to your body!

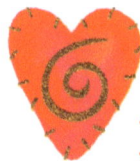

"To love oneself is the beginning of a lifelong romance." Oscar Wilde

The purpose of your wonderful rotator cuff is to center the head of the humerus in the center of your shoulder socket (glenoid) and **maintain** this position during any activities … such as pushing, pulling and throwing.

In order for you to have healthy shoulders that allow you to meet all the demands of your life your program must include exercises that:

- Maintain the proper alignment of the joint
- Strengthen the scapulae stabilizers and rotator cuff muscles (supraspinatus, infraspinatus, teres minor, subscapularis)
- Stretch the overly-facilitated, locked-short (tight) muscles such as pec major and lats

It is possible to have strong rotator cuff muscles while at the same time, have improper positioning (centration) of the head of the humerus. If your rotator cuff exercises are performed incorrectly, you may be creating or exaggerating the problem.

Anterior glide syndrome - a common problem:

Anterior humeral glide is when the upper portion of the humerus moves forward in relation to the shoulder socket itself especially with pushing or pulling movements. When this small little movement happens, it's usually the result of a cluster of things pushing it in this direction: the scapulae is in a position where it's tipped forward versus sitting flat to the rib cage; rounded shoulders; flexed thoracic spine; overuse of the upper traps. Serratus anterior, lower traps and rhomboids combine to help produce much of the scapulae stability for big movements, so if one or two aren't pulling their weight, the shoulder blade will wind up in a new position to accomplish the goal of lifting, pulling and pushing

A caveat here: it's difficult to make a definite diagnosis of anterior glide syndrome because the pain mimics many of the trigger point referral patterns of the rotator cuff and associated muscles. One symptom that is the most common is tenderness in the anterior shoulder and the posterior rotator cuff that does not resolve. I think it's a fair assumption that we all have a bit of it and the following exercises help with prevent and resolve it.

"IT DOES NOT MATTER HOW SLOWLY YOU GO SO LONG AS LONG AS YOU DO NOT STOP" (CONFUCIUS)

HUMERAL CENTRATION

Let's start with an easy/quick shoulder centration exercise so we teach the cuff to maintain proper positioning of the humeral head.

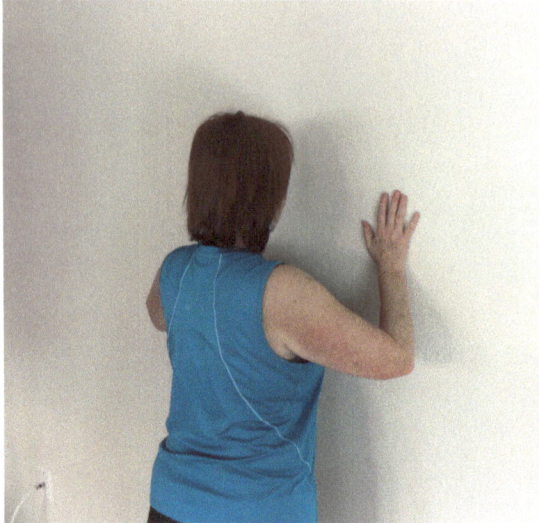

Step One:
- Position your hands on a wall.
- Place forearms on the wall.
- Slide the scapulae towards the lower back to anchor it

Step Two:
- Keeping the right hand and forearm on the wall, rotate to the left.
- Repeat on opposite side.
- Do 5-10 reps each side

The work is being done by the **stationary** arm by keeping the head of the humerus centrated.

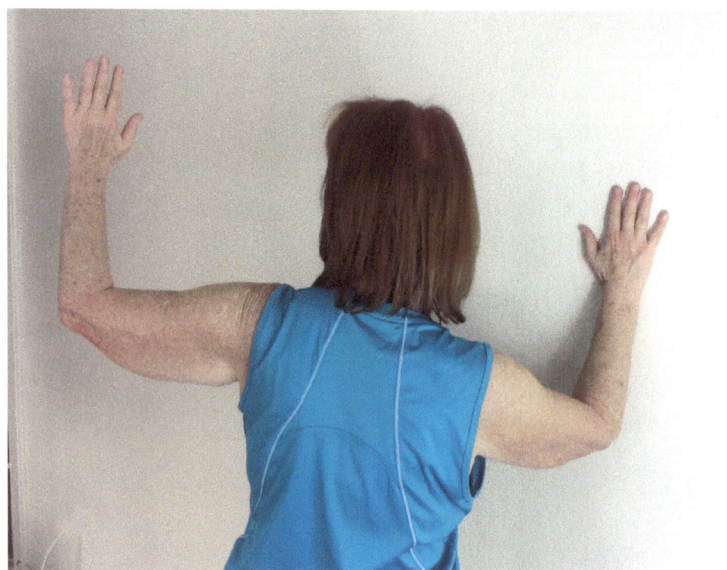

SELF-STRETCHES

Stretching the muscles that internally (rolls the shoulder forward) rotate is an absolute must for regaining a healthy balance between internal and external (rolls the shoulder backward) rotators of the shoulder joint and for good posture. Muscles that have been locked-short will not allow you to find an optimal posture and alignment of joints. Slow, gentle stretching re-educates these muscles. Most of the stretches on the following pages aim at opening the front of the body which has the added benefit of deepening the breath.

All stretches should be held for at least 15 seconds or longer - 3-4 deep breaths. Discontinue if the stretch causes or increases pain.

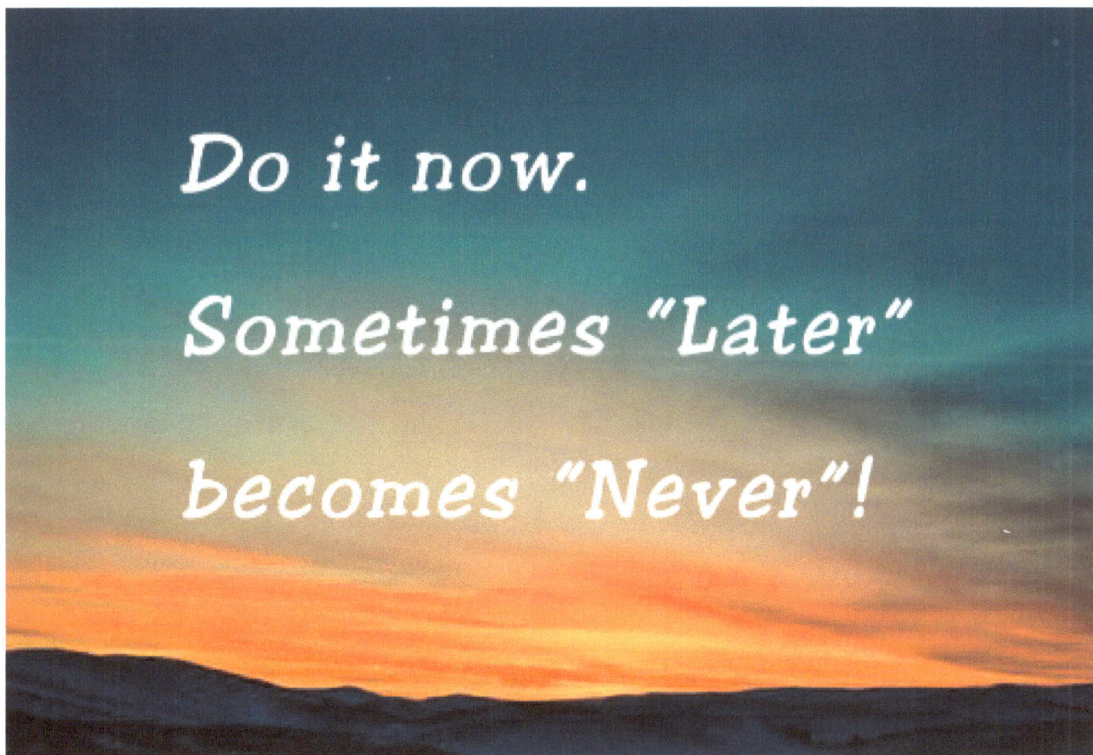

Do it now.

Sometimes "Later"

becomes "Never"!

SELF-STRETCHES

WALL STRETCH:

This is an easy stretch that can be done anywhere there is a wall! I recommend it as a starting stretch because you can easily control the intensity since it's one arm at a time.

• Start by placing your bent elbow against a wall.

• The humerus is lifted away from your side to shoulder level (shown) or higher. If you can't raise your arm to shoulder level, raise it to where you can with no pain and work from there.

• Leaving the elbow in place, turn your body, including your feet, away from your elbow.

• Hold and repeat on the other side.

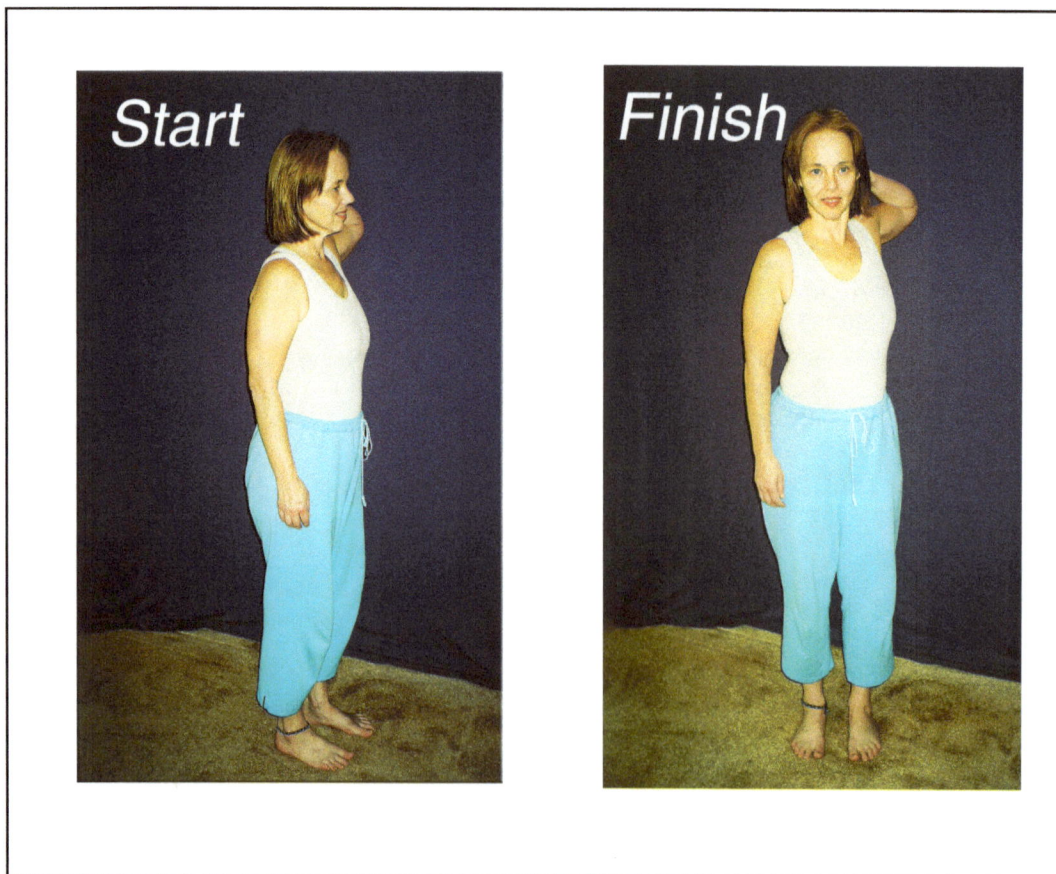

Errors to avoid:

■   Internally rotating the shoulder joint. Maintain external rotation.

■   Walking the feet away from the wall. Keep the body in a straight "column."

SELF-STRETCHES

THORACIC SPINE MOBILITY EXERCISE

Your thoracic spine is the middle section of your vertebra between your neck and lower back and is comprised of 12 thoracic vertebras and your rib cage. Thoracic mobility involves available movement of this portion of the spine and is very important for achieving or maintaining good posture. Thoracic spine mobility is an extremely important, and often times overlooked, component to a variety of dysfunctions. Poor thoracic mobility can affect the shoulder, neck, low back, and hip very easily. Unfortunately, our daily habits and posture make us all very prone to poor thoracic spine mobility.

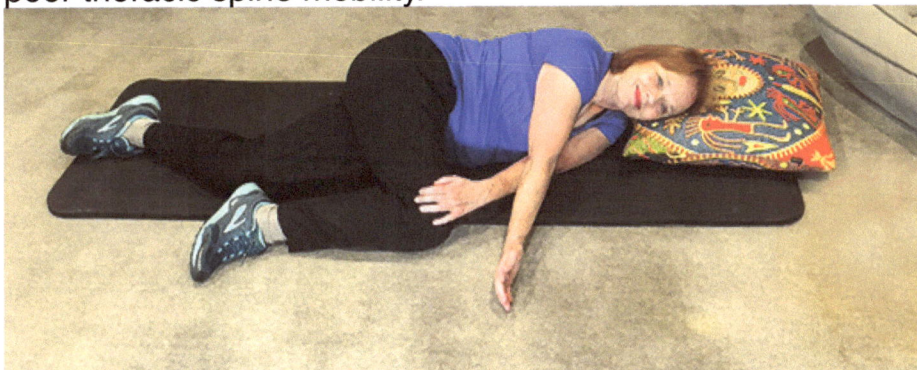

Step One:
- Lie on your side with your head supported by a pillow. Your bottom leg is straight. Your top leg is bent.
- Place the palm of your lower (the side you are lying on) hand on the knee of your top leg. Maintain that hand placement during the exercise.
- Place your top hand pinky down on the floor

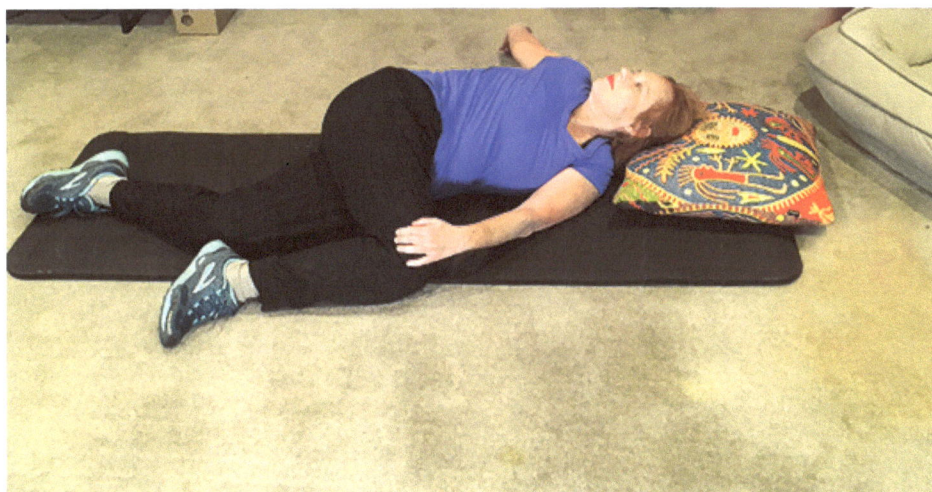

Step Two:
- Reach your top arm behind you, shoulder height and keep your palm up
- Allow your eyes to follow your hand.
- If your arm does not contact the floor, no problem! Don't force it - it will come in time. Do 5-10 reps each side.

OVER THE SMALL BALL STRETCH:

This is a wonderful self-stretch for stretching and opening the chest, and increasing spinal mobility. It's a personal favorite of mine - I start and end my days with it. It requires a ball about the size of the one below. The ball needs to be soft enough so it's comfortable.

Place the ball under the *mid-back* so the head is supported by the floor. Make sure to bend the knees with the feet flat on the floor to create a neutral pelvis and protect the low back. Hold for as long as it's comfortable.

If you have limited flexibility, start with the pillow stretch on the next page.

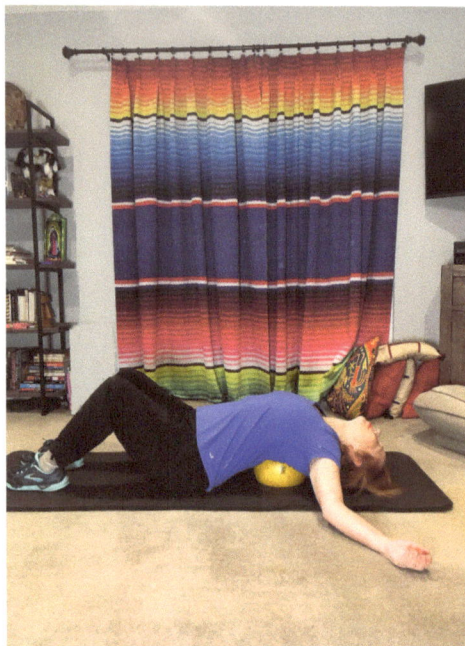

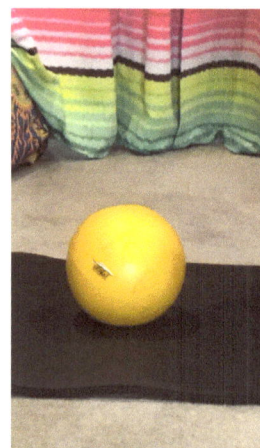

OVER THE BIG BALL STRETCH:

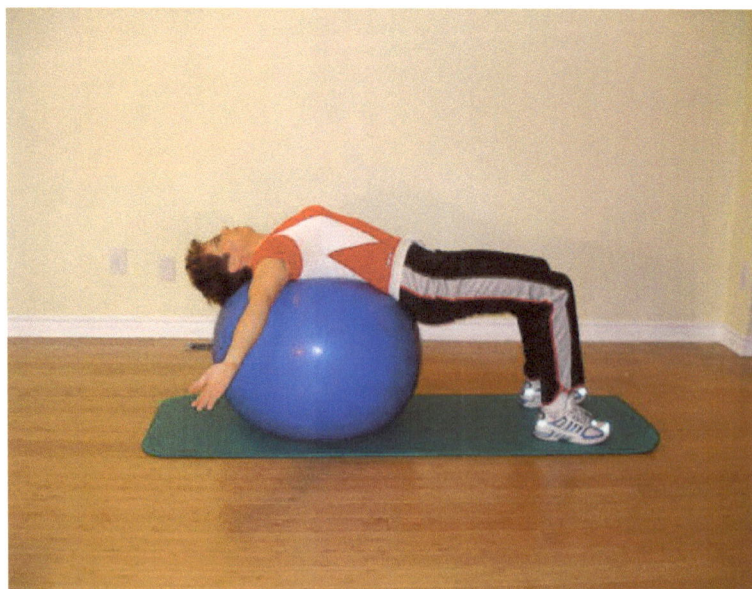

- Lie back over the exercise ball with the ball centered under your thoracic spine.

- Allow your back to gently arch over the ball.

- Reach arms overhead or to the side. To make the stretch more intense allow the elbows to straighten. Less intense: bend your elbows.

- Hold this position for as long it's comfortable. Enjoy!

Over the pillow stretch:

This is a wonderful self-stretch for the internal rotators that can be done alone or assisted. It feels marvelous! Prop one or more pillows under the *mid-back* so the head is supported by the bed or floor. The number of pillows depends on your flexibility. If you have limited flexibility, start with one pillow and build up. Make sure the shoulders are rolled back in external rotation. **The arms can be over the head or out to the side, depending on flexibility.** This stretch is also great for deepening the breath and has the added benefit of gently increasing spinal flexibility. Make sure to bend the knees with the feet flat on the floor to create a neutral pelvis and protect the low back.

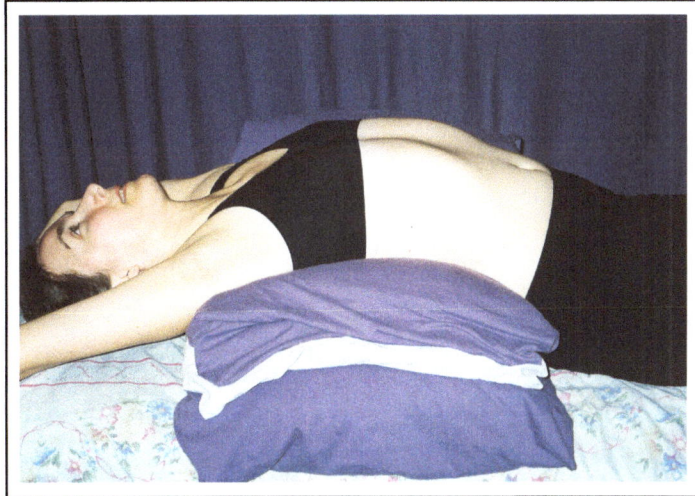

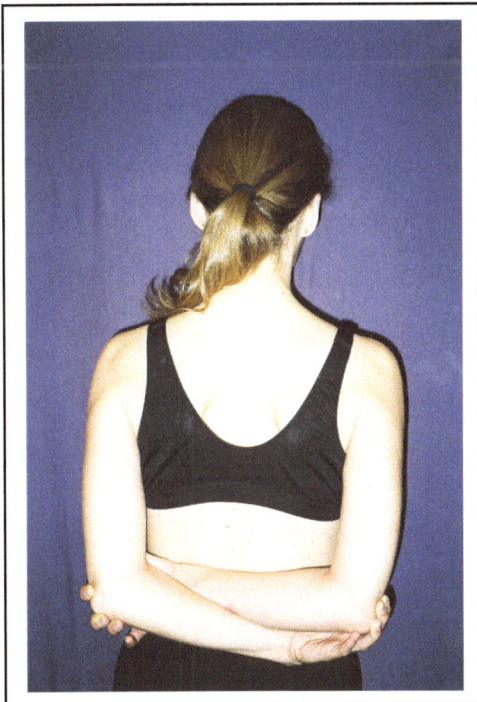

Cradle the arms behind you stretch:

This is an excellent and gentle self-stretch for the muscles that roll the shoulder joint forward in internal rotation that can be done as many times during the day as possible, especially for someone who works at a computer. Cradle the arms behind by grasping the forearms or elbows; then squeeze the shoulder blades together.

*This stretch is only for those who can bring their arms behind the back with no pain.

38

BAND STRETCH: This stretch can be done with a towel, scarf, or belt. *This stretch is only for those who can raise their arms overhead with no pain.

•Place your hands on either end of whatever you are using and lift your arms up over your head.

•Shrug your shoulders up, then let them fall down.

•*Level One:* slowly press your arms back, keeping the elbows straight but not locked. Hold for at least fifteen seconds.

•*Level Two:* for a more intense stretch (not recommended for the early stages of recovery), bring the arms down behind the back, then back up to starting position. Repeat 3 to 5 reps.

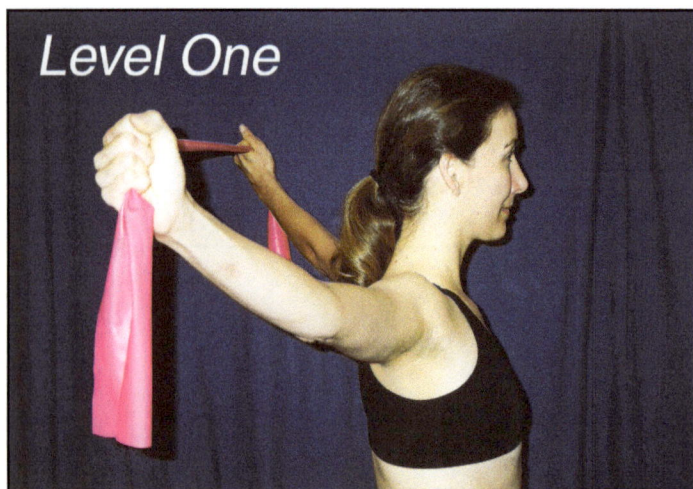

Level One

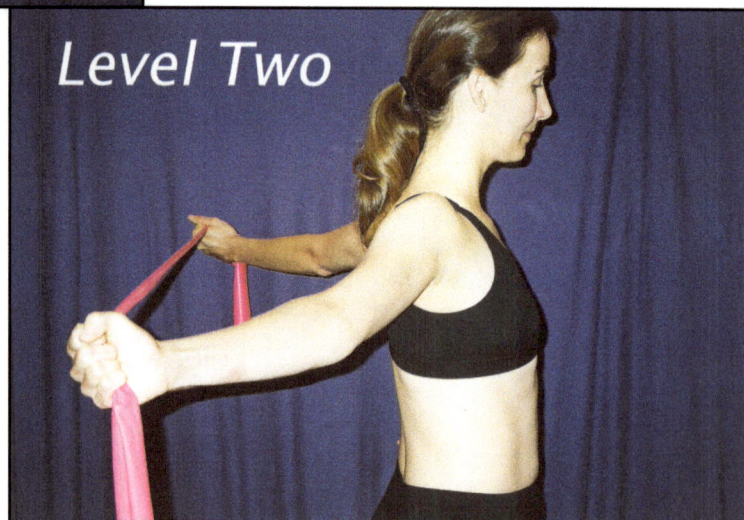

Level Two

Errors to avoid:

■   Internally rotating the shoulder joint. Maintain external rotation.
■   Allowing the pelvis to tip forward. Maintain neutral lumbar alignment.

SELF-STRETCHES

STANDING SHOULDER STRETCH:

This is a great stretch for the big latissimus dorsi muscle which is not only important for shoulder health but also for low back and SI joint health. This versatile stretch can be done on a bannister (shown), a dining room table, a chair or an exercise ball (shown). The instructions apply to whatever surface you choose. In the bannister photos, the left side is shown. In the ball photos the right side is shown.

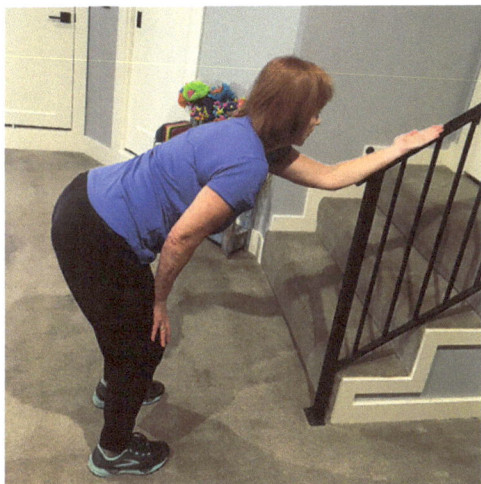

Step One: Stand behind the surface and place your left hand palm up. Place your right hand palm down over your left hand.

Step Two: While maintaining a neutral lumbar spine (don't let your back arch or your pelvis to tuck under) twist your spine to your right until you feel just the right amount of stretch on the left side. Hold for 15-30 seconds and repeat on the other side.

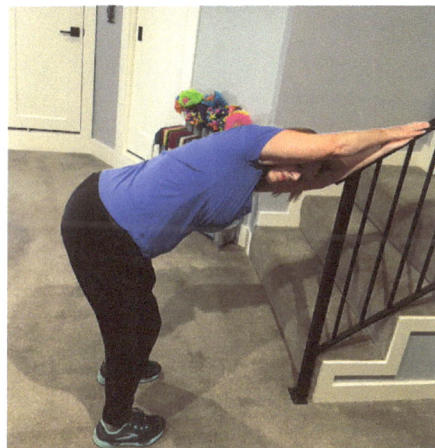

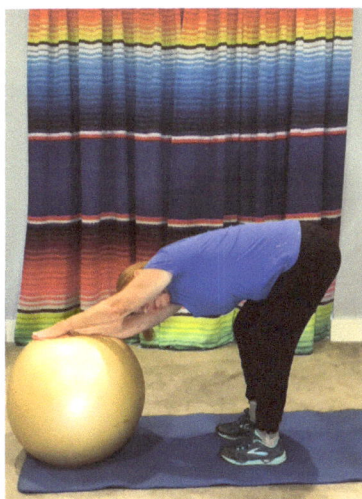

Photo left: The right hand is palm down and the body twists to the left to stretch the right side.

BROOMSTICK STRETCH:

This is a great stretch that targets Muscle #4 (subscapularis) which always needs lengthening. The photos below show the left Muscle #4 being stretched.

• Place a broomstick behind the back, grasp the pole end with the left hand, palm facing out with the humerus lifted away from your side to shoulder height.
• The right hand gently pushes the broom end forward which increases the degree of external rotation. Hold for at least fifteen seconds.
• To stretch the right Muscle #4, reverse the instructions. Maintain neutral alignment of the spine.

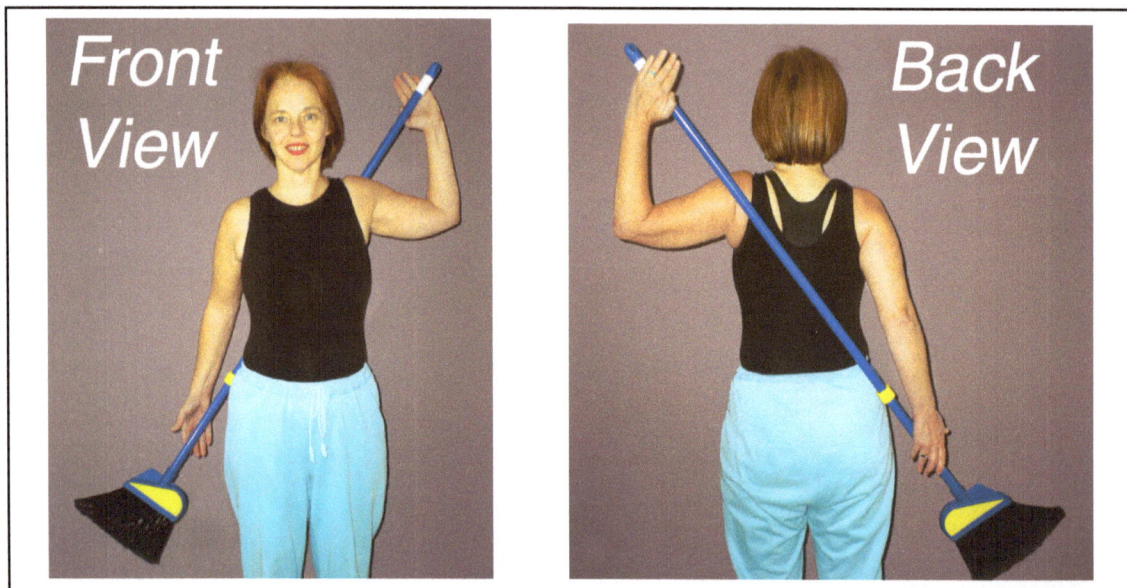

MUSCLE #1 STRETCH (SUPRASPINATUS):

Grasp the forearm of the side you want to stretch and slowly pull it across the back. The photo right shows the left Muscle #1 being stretched.

Errors to avoid:

■   Internally rotating the shoulder joint.
■   Bending your torso to the side. Maintain upright posture.

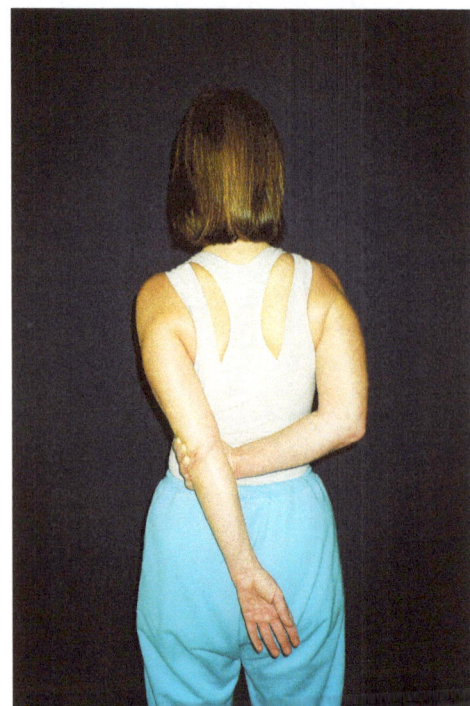

Strengthening Exercises

The scapula (shoulder blade) plays a critical role in maintaining shoulder joint function. The scapula is the base of support for all shoulder joint and upper quadrant movements.

Think of the scapula as the core of your upper body or the foundation of your house. A strong shoulder core allows for greater distal* strength: Putting a suitcase in the overhead compartment of an airplane or playing racket sports. The stronger the scapular stabilizers the less load is put on the weaker muscles of the extremities.

Poor stabilization can contribute to a wide variety of problems such as impingement, rotator cuff tears, cervical strain, nerve entrapment's and problems in the forearm such as tennis and golfers elbow.

Let's work to improve the stabilization of our scapulae so we can enjoy our work, our families and our leisure activities.

In the next couple of exercises we'll be working on strengthening the large scapular stabilizers, primarily serratus anterior, middle and lower traps, rhomboids and latissimus dorsi/teres major. These exercises also help with humeral centration.

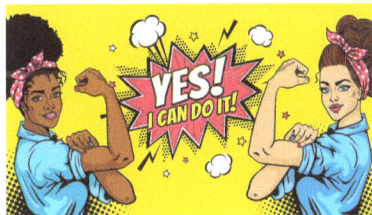

Parts of the body further away from the center. For example, the hand is distal to the shoulder. The thumb is distal to the wrist.

SCAPULAE STABILIZATION EXERCISES

Here's a quick and easy exercise you can do when you take those all important breaks from a computer that activate the scapulae stabilizers:

As you are doing this exercise imagine that you are putting your shoulder blades into your back pockets.

"WALK TO THE WALL"

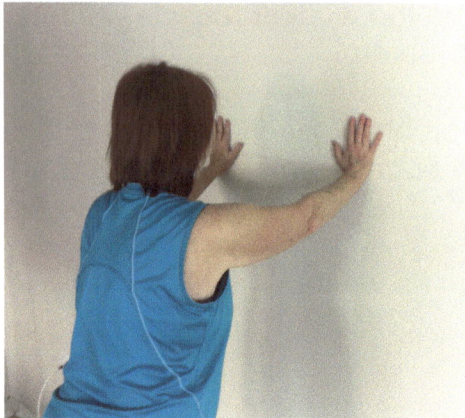

Step One:
- Position your hands about two feet away from a wall.
- Your arms are shoulder width apart.

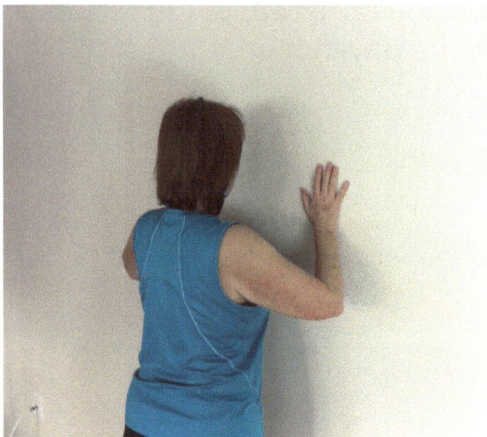

Step Two:
- Walk to the wall.
- Place forearms on wall

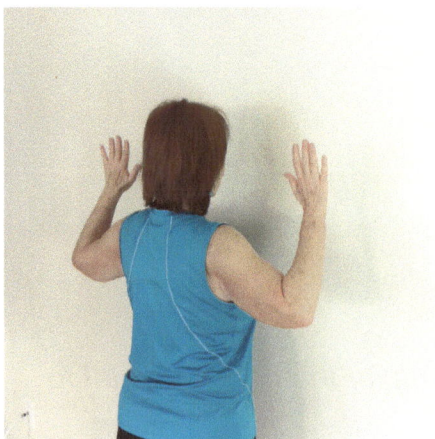

Step Three:
- Lift your hands off the wall. You should feel an immediate activation of the scapulae retractors: rhomboids and middle traps.
- Do 5-10 reps

SCAPULAE STABILIZATION EXERCISES

Here's a another quick and easy exercise you can do that's especially good for the serratus anterior, a muscle that plays a key role in stabilizing your scapulae. I like to do a couple of these between clients.

"PUSH THE TOWEL"
Roll a towel like the one pictured. Place rubber bands around the end so it stays in position.

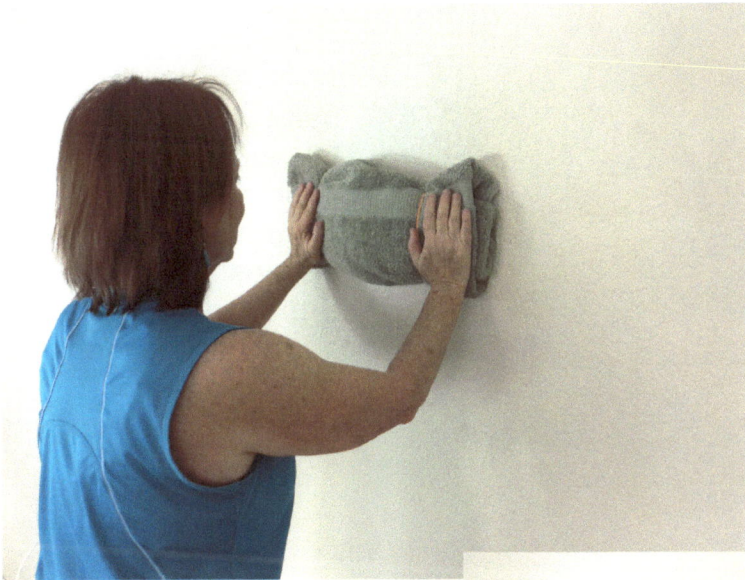

Step One:
- Position your hands on the towel about a foot away from a wall.
- Your arms are shoulder width apart.

Step Two:
- Slide the towel up the wall.
- Shift your weight to the balls of your feet and allow the body to lean in maintaining alignment
- Slide the towel down the wall and return to neutral.
- Do 5-10 reps

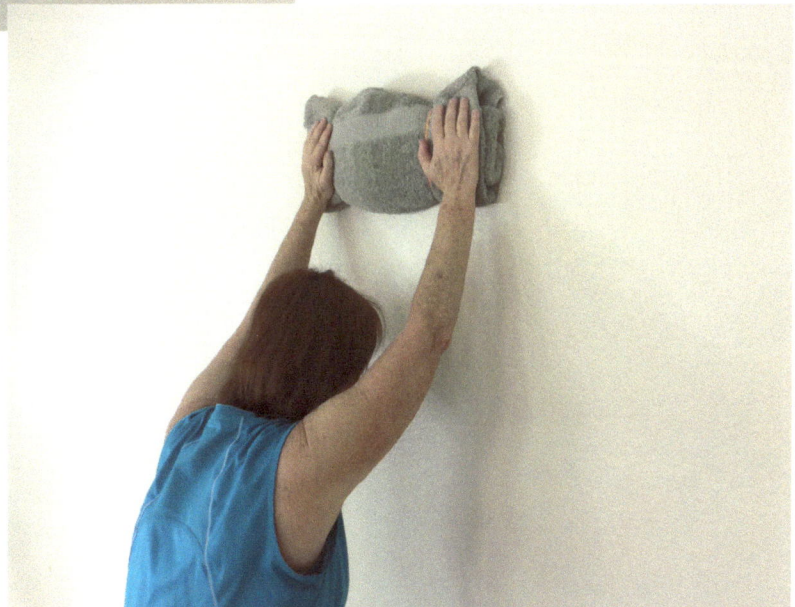

TIP: Imagine you have magnets attached to your inner elbows drawing them towards each other. This prevents the elbows from moving away from the body.

SCAPULAE STABILIZATION EXERCISES

V's and T's are staples in activating and strengthening the scapulae stabilizers:

As you are doing this exercise imagine you are putting your shoulder blades into your back pockets.

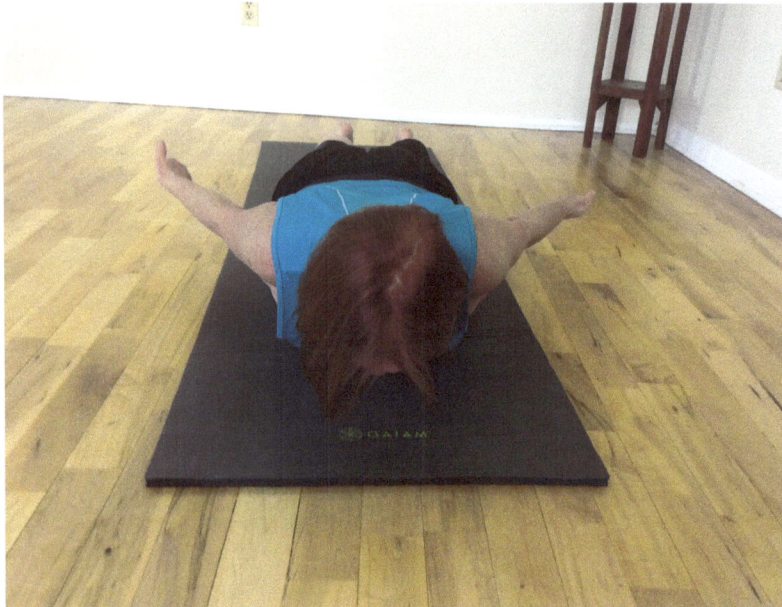

V's:

- Lie prone on a mat.
- Slightly tuck your tailbone to protect the low back
- Arms are at your side palm down
- Lift your arms off the floor. Externally rotate the shoulder joint so the thumbs are up
- Squeeze a hundred dollar bill between your shoulder blades!
- Hold for 15-20 seconds
- Do 5-10 reps

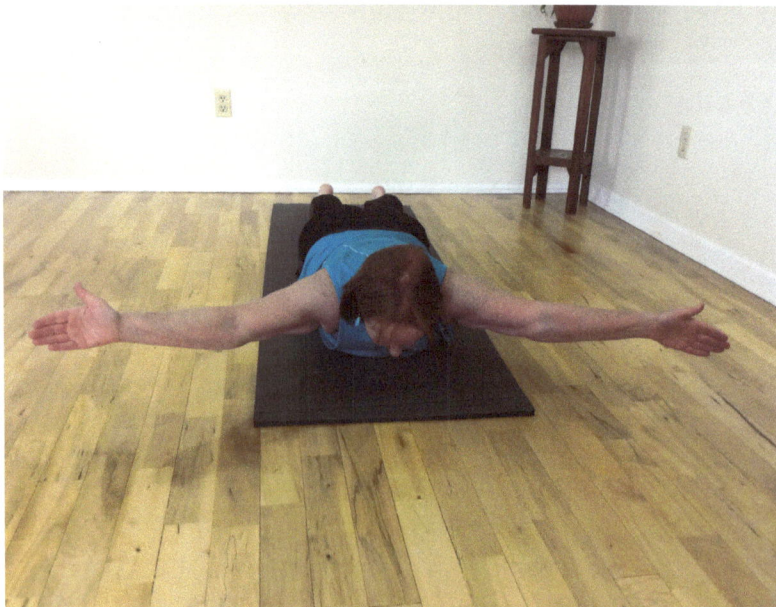

T's:

- Lie prone on a mat.
- Slightly tuck your tailbone to protect the low back
- Arms are away from your side palm down
- Lift your arms off the floor. Externally rotate the shoulder joint so the thumbs are up
- Squeeze a hundred dollar bill between your shoulder blades!
- Hold for 15-20 seconds
- Do 5-10 reps

The following exercises are done on an exercise ball which is a great tool for both strengthening and stretching. Balls are available on the web, and at most sporting goods stores.

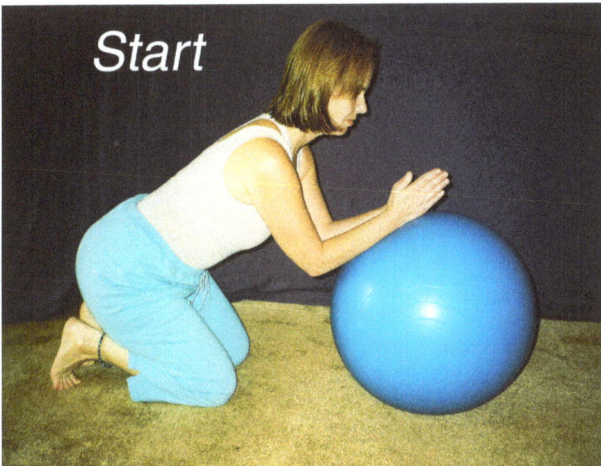

Start

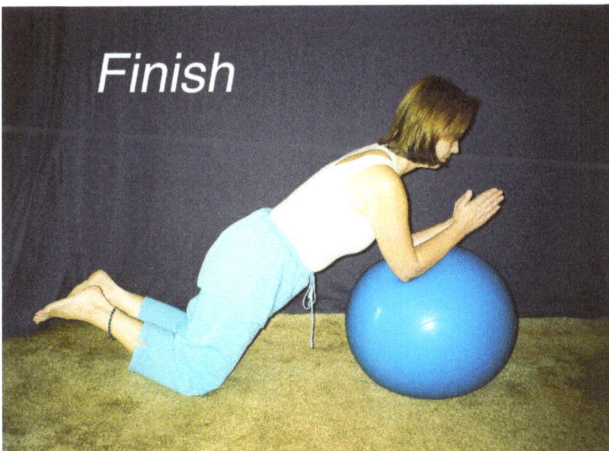

Finish

FORWARD ROLL:

Starting position: kneeling on the floor with the palms together as if praying. The hands should be on the part of the ball nearest to your body.

• Gently retract the shoulder blades (squeeze them together) and from this "altar boy" position, roll forward until your elbows rest atop the ball.
• Lift your toes off the floor.
• Roll only far enough to feel the shoulder girdle muscles engage. Rolling too far will target the abdominals. You want to make certain you feel it more in the shoulder girdle.
• Maintaining neutral position of the lumbar and cervical spine, keep your hips extended throughout the exercise.
• See that the hips are in line with spine and not hiked upward.
• This is an excellent isometric exercise for strengthening the stabilizing muscles of both the shoulder joint and shoulder girdle. Hold for ten seconds to start and build up to one minute.

As you are doing this exercise imagine you are putting your shoulder blades into your back pockets and squeeze your elbows together.

SUPERPERSON:

Starting position: prone position with trunk support, knees off the floor. Your hands rest lightly on the floor. Light dumbbells may be held to make this exercise more intense.

- Maintaining neutral position of the lumbar and cervical spine, squeeze your shoulder blades together.
- Then slowly lift your arms directly up until your hands are approximately at shoulder height.
- Pause at the top of the movement, hold for 15 seconds, then slowly lower the arms to starting position and repeat.
- Maintain shoulder blade retraction throughout the exercise, releasing upon return to starting position. The shoulder blade retraction stabilizes the shoulder girdle prior to the movement.
- Do not allow the spine to arch or the chest to lift off the ball as you raise your arms.

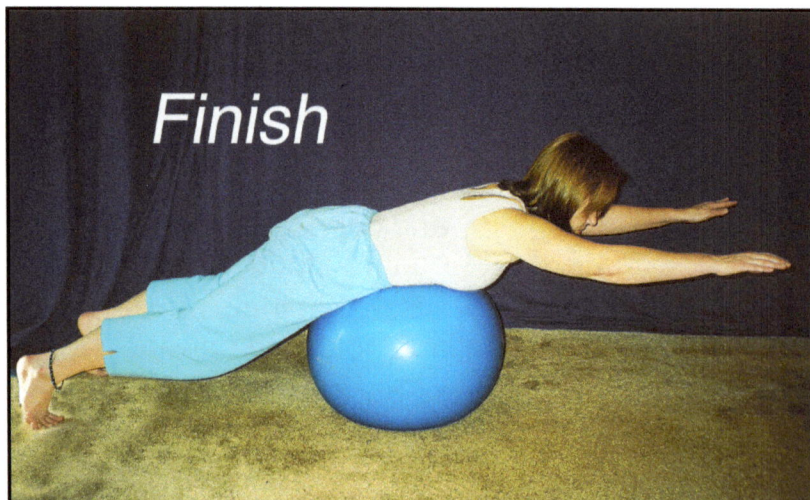

Finish

As you are doing this exercise imagine you are putting your shoulder blades into your back pockets.

STRENGTHENING EXTERNAL ROTATORS

The following exercises are useful for strengthening the muscles of the rotator cuff and shoulder girdle that tend to be weak. Go slowly, respect your body's pain tolerance and remember that often with injuries, *less is more*.

STRENGTHENING EXERCISES FOR MUSCLES # 2 AND 3
(INFRASPINATUS AND TERES MINOR):

"THE FLASHER": This is a good beginning exercise.

• Using a light or medium weight resistance band bend the elbows and "glue" them to the waist.

• Separate the forearms as if you were opening both sides of a coat.

• Slowly return to starting position. The return trip provides what's called eccentric strengthening or working the negative. Most injuries to these muscles occur from being over-stretched, so gradual strengthening on the return is a good preventative.

• Start with three sets of five repetitions and gradually increase to ten repetitions.

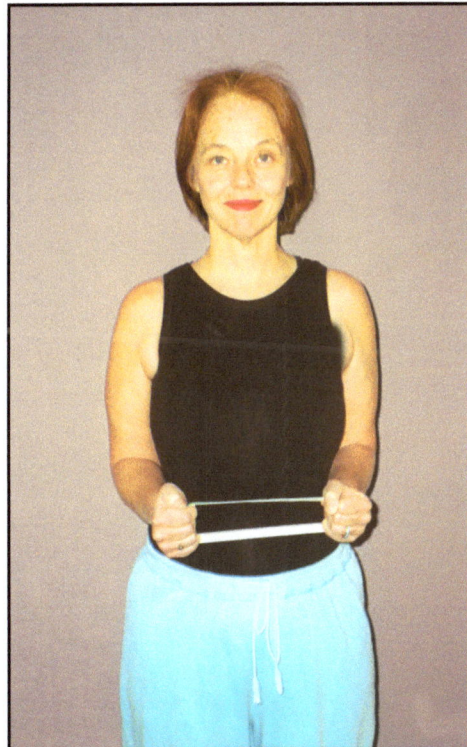

Errors to avoid:

■ Leading with the wrists. The wrists should remain in neutral position.
■ Increasing the bend in the elbow as you separate the forearms. Maintain a 90 degree bend.
■ Letting the elbows come away from the body. Make sure they stay "glued" to the waist.

LYING "L" FLYES:

This is a more difficult exercise and can be started when you can easily do "The Flasher" without pain. Using a 1 to 5 pound weight (no more than a five pound weight; even a can of soup can be used!); do three sets of 5-10 repetitions. Lie on your side with the head either supported by your hand or resting on your arm.

• Place your elbow on the waist at a 90 degree angle (you can place a towel under your elbow for support).

• Make sure the elbow stays "glued" to the waist as you externally rotate the humerus and raise your hand up toward the ceiling, maintaining the 90 degree bend in the elbow and keeping the wrist in neutral. Slowly return to the middle of the movement range. Most injuries to these muscles occur from being over-stretched so gradual strengthening on the return is a good preventative. This eccentric part of the exercise is the most important.

• Hold at this halfway point for 10 seconds for isometric/stabilizing strengthening. Return to starting position. Repeat on other side to insure muscle balance on both shoulders.

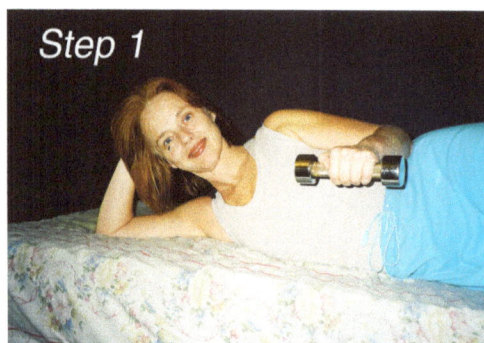

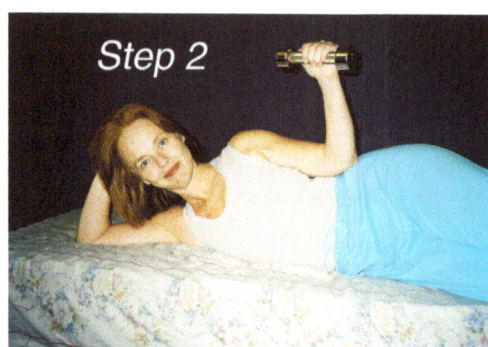

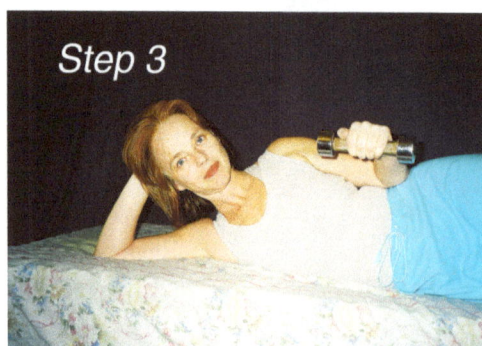

Errors to avoid:

- ■ Raising the humerus off your body while performing the exercise. Imagine that the humerus and elbow are "glued" to your side.
- ■ Increasing the bend in the elbow as you externally rotate. Maintain a 90 degree bend.
- ■ Rolling back as you perform the exercise. Keep the upper body in the same plane during the exercise.

STRENGTHENING SCAPULAE RETRACTORS

PULL BACKS: Primary muscles worked: middle and lower trapezius, rhomboids.

•Grasp a resistance band palms facing down.

•Hold the band about six inches from your torso at the height of the lowest part of your chest bone

•Squeeze the shoulder blades together. Hold for ten seconds.

 •Your goal is not to stretch the band apart. The band provides just the right amount of resistance so your muscles have to work a wee bit harder.

•Repeat with three sets of five to start, building up to ten repetitions.

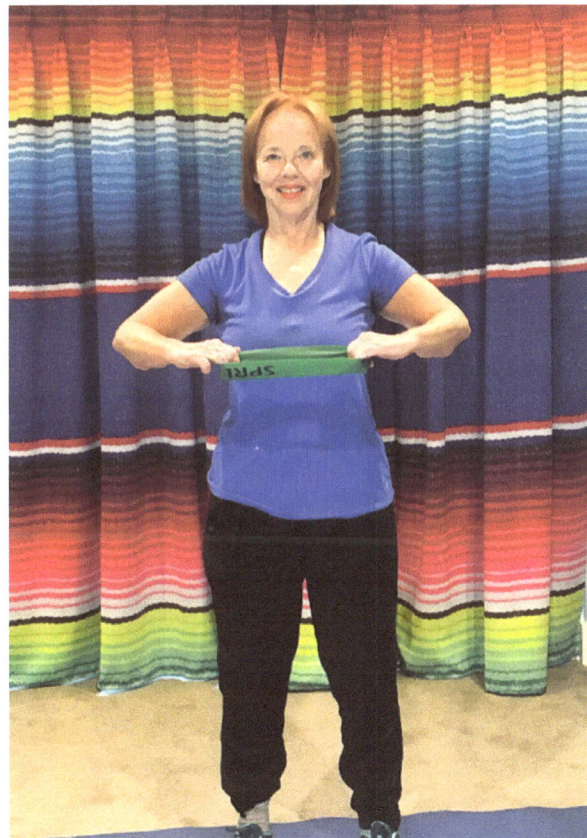

Need a medium resistance band? Click on the link below. Use coupon code VBNGCVD2 at checkout for a $3 discount. Your price - only $7

www.massagepublications. com/product/exercise-bands

Errors to avoid:

■ Jutting the chin and neck forward. Maintain proper neck alignment.
■ Allowing the shoulders to rise. Let them to stay in neutral position.
■ Allowing the pelvis to tilt forward or backward. Maintain proper low back alignment.

PULL DOWNS:*

*This exercise is only for those who can raise their arms overhead with no pain.
*People who have been diagnosed with anterior capsule problems should avoid this exercise.

• Grasp a resistance band, palms facing out, arms overhead.

• Squeeze the shoulder blades together, pull the band apart, lower the arms to behind the middle of the head, or shoulder level.

• Hold for 10 seconds.

• Start with three sets of five repetitions and build up to ten repetitions.

• This is a great exercise to bring the torso into alignment with the pelvis but you'll need to pay attention to neck alignment - don't allow the chin and neck to jut forward. This exercise has the added benefit of stretching the internal rotators, especially the pectoralis major.

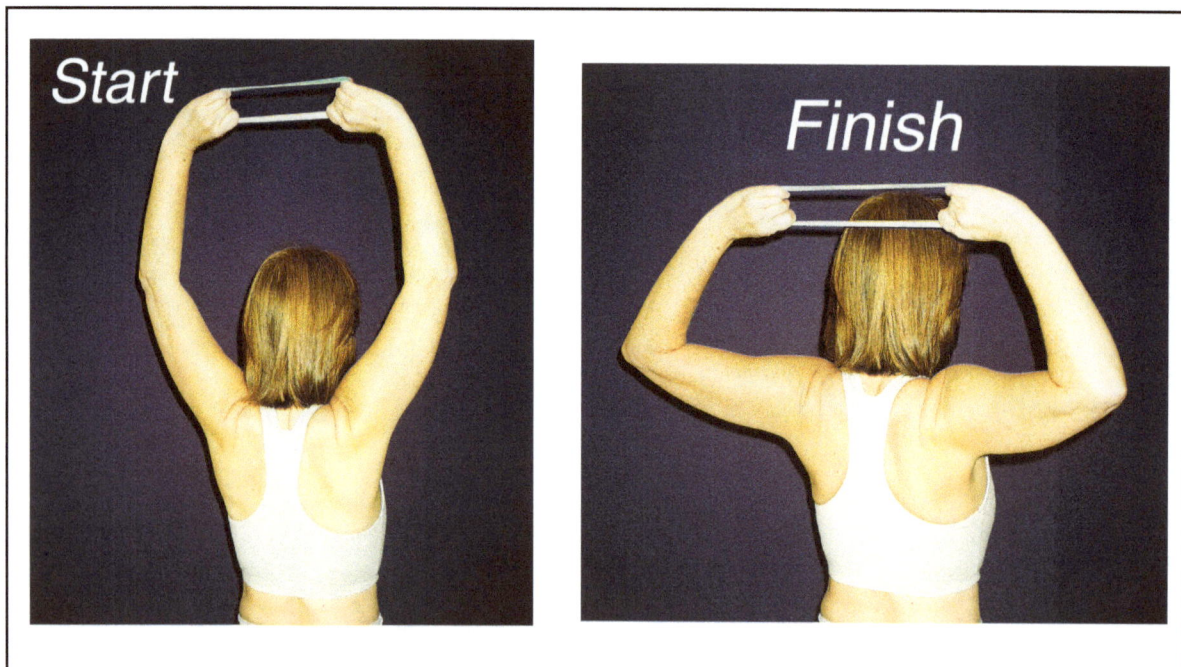

Start

Finish

Errors to avoid:

■   Jutting the chin and neck forward. Maintain proper cervical alignment.
■   Allowing the shoulders to rise. Let them to stay in neutral position.
■   Allowing the pelvis to tilt forward or backward. Maintain proper low back alignment.

Sample Routines

Take care of
your body -
it's the only
place you have
to live!

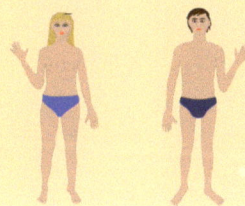

SAMPLE ROUTINES

A reminder: shoulder problems can be complex, multidimensional and multifaceted. This booklet is not a comprehensive study of those issues. This manual is for educational purposes only and should not be considered a substitute for proper training. It is sold with the understanding that the author and publisher are not engaged in rendering medical or other professional services. If medical advice or other expert assistance is required, the services of an appropriate professional should be sought. Information in this book should not be used to diagnose, treat, or prescribe. The author and publisher shall not be held liable for any damages in connection with, or arising out of anyone's interpretation or application of the information in this manual. The user is encouraged to always use sound judgment in making decisions about her/his ability to perform the exercises.

If any of these exercises makes your problem worse, STOP! Consult an appropriate medical professional....

That being said, below are a couple of sample routines. Listen to your body and add to or subtract to create a routine that works for you.

I HAVE ISSUES! WHERE SHOULD I START?

1. Humeral Centration: 5x each side
2. Pendulum: 3x per day; 3-5 minutes each set
3. Thoracic Spine Mobility: 5x each side
4. Push the towel: 5x
5. Walk to the Wall: 5x
6. One Pec Stretch

All of the above three times a week.
This routine only takes ten minutes and you can do as a group or break it up. This is also a great routine whether you have shoulder issues or not.

INTERMEDIATE/ADVANCED AND/OR MY SHOULDERS ARE IN GOOD SHAPE AND I WANT TO KEEP THEM THAT WAY!

1. Humeral Centration: 10 reps each side
2. Thoracic Spine Mobility: 10x each side
3. V's: 10 reps
4. V's: 10 reps
5. You can alternate the V's and T's with the Forward Roll and Superwoman on an exercise ball
6. The flasher or Lying L Flyes: 10 reps
7. Pull downs or Pull backs: 10 reps
8. Broomstick Stretch
9. Supraspinatus Stretch
10. One (or more) Pec Stretch
11. Standing Shoulder Stretch

All of the above three times a week.
This routine only takes about 20 minutes and you can do as a group or break it up.

End your day with a yummy Over the Ball or Pillow stretch and deep breathing!

VISUALIZATIONS FOR HAPPY MOVEMENT

If we look at rotator cuff injuries globally, we find that incorrect body mechanics and movement contribute to this condition. Good posture and movement are essential to a vibrant, healthy and enjoyable life. To consistently ignore our body requires enormous repressive energies. To learn more about our body, to use it more efficiently and for more activities requires constant attention to the creation of new movements and the novel sensations they bring.

Movement allows us to feel alive, vital and passionate about life. When we move in a variety of ways, different parts of our nervous system are stimulated, giving us a new sense of ourselves, a fresh identity. The visualizations below are ones that I've collected from many sources to encourage a new and happy sense of movement.

♦   *Imagine you have a feather attached vertically at the back of your head. As you move your head let the feather draw shapes in the sky.*

♦   *Visualize your neck as an incredibly long, golden, flexible coil of taffy that can move effortlessly in many directions. Discover where your coil can go and cannot go. Feel the pliability and agility as they increase in your neck.*

♦   *Imagine the skull as a big vertebra sitting on top of the spine.*

♦   *Imagine that your arms are beautiful white wings. As you move them, feel the wind lifting and lowering your arms.*

♦   *As you inhale deeply, feel your ribs expanding to the sides of the room, gently touching the walls. At the same time, experience and visualize the lengthening of your spine as if it were an elegant redwood tree extending high into the sky.*

♦   *Visualize your breath as having a color. See that color of breath filling up your entire chest, horizontally and vertically as you inhale. Sense your clavicles being gently widened by the breath color inside you.*

♦   *As you inhale and exhale, visualize your ribs moving like an accordion as your lungs expand and contract. The accordion closes on the exhale and opens on the inhale. Enjoy the stretch from inside.*

♦   *Create more range of motion at the sternoclavicular joint by imagining the clavicles opening and widening out into space.*

♦   *Imagine a flower in the center of your chest. As you inhale, let the flower open up farther and farther until you can smell the fragrance.*

HAPPY EXPLORATIONS!

Index

Peggy Lamb will tell you she is a massage therapist. She is a massage therapist, but she is so much more than that. When Peggy confronts a problem, she doesn't just solve the problem for herself. She will solve the problem for others, and try to insure that the problem isn't a problem for all her clients. When she tore a rotator cuff, she learned about shoulders, about how they move, how the function, and how they function well. Not only did she completely recover from her injury, she wrote a book "Releasing the Rotator Cuff" so other massage therapists can help their clients with shoulder injuries. When faced with a back injury, Peggy worked to recover from that, and recover she did. Not content to just overcome her own injury, she wrote another book "The Core of the Matter", with content geared to help others, and other massage therapists, with back problems. Peggy doesn't just fix issues that come up in her life, but she resolves those issues for others. Peggy Lamb is not just a massage therapist, she is an author of five books, a creator of four instructional DVDs, a teacher of massage therapists, a leader in her field. All of this comes from one feeling…..the desire to touch, to heal, and to be touched.

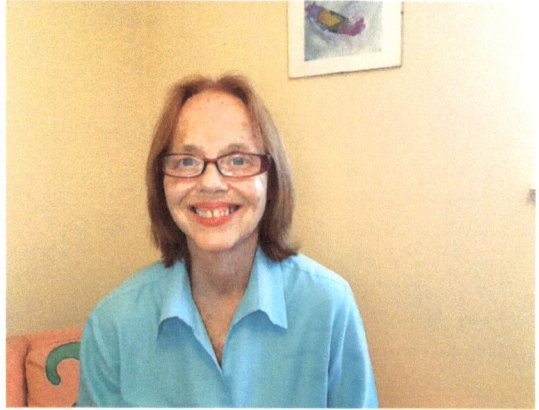